THE
REBIRTH
OF THE
CLINIC

Praise for *The Rebirth of the Clinic*

"A collection of heartfelt, insightful, avowedly confessional essays by a respected physician-ethicist who is a powerful spokesperson both for Roman Catholic views of health and medicine and for a consideration of spirituality in clinician/patient interactions."

—Margaret Mohrmann, M.D., Ph.D., University of Virginia

"Sulmasy builds a scholarly foundation for spirituality as the essential element for good health care practice. Weaving historically derived insights with scholarly investigation and critical thought, Dr. Sulmasy convincingly establishes the case that all health care professionals have the moral obligation to attend to the human spirit in the healing encounter. [*The Rebirth of the Clinic*] is the resource health care professionals can use to reclaim the heart and humanity of medicine."

—Christina M. Puchalski, M.D., director, The George
Washington Institute for Spirituality and Health

"This book joins others which grapple with the meaning of caring for the dying, but it adds to them by its depth of understanding and its focus on religion and spirituality. . . . Sulmasy is one of few true visionaries, scholars and critics of the intersection of religion, spirituality and medicine."

—Farr Curlin, M.D., The University of Chicago

"Sulmasy's insight, intellect, and spirituality have produced a superb philosophy of medicine and theology of the transcendent. This excellent foundational work is given a remarkably practical application by his bedside experience in the practice of medicine."

—Robert D. Orr, M.D., C.M., University of Vermont College of
Medicine

"One of those rare works that nourishes the mind, heart, and soul. Readers will be challenged intellectually but also invited to experience the profundity of the healer–patient encounter . . . a truly remarkable achievement."

—Mark G. Kuczewski, director, The Neiswanger Institute for
Bioethics & Health Policy, Loyola University Chicago

THE
REBIRTH
OF THE
CLINIC

An Introduction to Spirituality in Health Care

Daniel P. Sulmasy, O.F.M., M.D.

GEORGETOWN UNIVERSITY PRESS
Washington, D.C.

As of January 1, 2007, 13-digit ISBN numbers will replace the current 10-digit system.
Paperback: 978-1-58901-095-6

Georgetown University Press, Washington, D.C.

Library of Congress Cataloging-in-Publication Data

Sulmasy, Daniel P., 1956–
    The rebirth of the clinic : an introduction to spirituality in health care /
Daniel P. Sulmasy.
        p.   cm.
    Includes bibliographical references and index.
    ISBN-13: 978-1-58901-095-6 (pbk. : alk. paper)
    ISBN-10: 1-58901-095-7 (pbk. : alk. paper)
    1. Medical care—Religious aspects.   2. Spirituality.   3. Terminal
care—Religious aspects.   I. Title.
    R725.55.S83   2006
    362.1—dc22   2005027250

This book is printed on acid-free paper meeting the requirements of the American
National Standard for Permanence in Paper for Printed Library Materials.

13 12 11 10 09 08 07 06   9 8 7 6 5 4 3 2
First printing

Printed in the United States of America

For my parents, whose example and teaching inspired me to lead the life of a Friar minor and a physician.

Contents

Acknowledgments   ix

Introduction   xi

Part I. Rebirth in the Clinic

1 Why Surgeons Must Be Very Careful   3

2 Is Health Care a Spiritual Practice?   13

3 Dignity, Vulnerability, and the Personhood of the Patient   24

4 The Wisdom of Ben Sira   44

5 The Dialectic of Healing   60

6 Taking Physicians' Oaths Seriously   89

**Part II. The Book of Numbers: Empirical Research on
           Spirituality and Healing**

7 What the Data Cannot Mean   115

8 A Biopsychosocial-Spiritual Model of Health Care   121

9 Scientific Studies of the Healing Power of Prayer   147

10 Is There a Moral Obligation to Address the Spiritual Needs
   of Patients?   161

Part III. At the Threshold of Death

11 On Praying for a Cure   189

12 Healing the Dying   197

13 At W;t's End   213

14 Peg   224

    Postscript: Is There Life after the Clinic?   237

    Index   239

Acknowledgments

B ooks do not just happen. They take time—an extremely precious commodity for a medical school professor. Books also are collegial efforts. This one could not have been written alone. Therefore I am deeply grateful to the Department of Theology at St. John's University, New York, where I was a visiting professor as Mc- Keever Chair in Moral Theology, 2003–2004, which enabled me to do most of the work that made this book possible. In particular, I would like to thank Dr. Sidney Callahan for suggesting my name to St. John's and Fr. Pat Primeaux, S.M., chair of the department. I owe a huge debt of gratitude to my colleague Lynn Jansen, RN, PhD, who ably picked up so many of my responsibilities at St. Vincent's Hospital–Manhattan and New York Medical College, enabling me to devote time to this book and other writing projects. I also am enormously grateful to Dr. Alan Astrow, a friend and fellow traveler in the fields of spirituality and health care, who read this entire manuscript and helped to edit this book. Finally, I am grateful to the anonymous reviewers for Georgetown University Press who made extremely insightful and useful comments.

All scriptural quotes, unless otherwise noted, are from the *New Revised Standard Version Bible* (New York: Division of Christian Education of the National Council of the Churches of Christ in the United States, 1989).

Several chapters in this book are based on work I have published previously. Where applicable, the current versions appear with permission:

- Chapter 2: "Is Medicine a Spiritual Practice?" *Academic Medicine* 74 (1999): 1002–5 (© 1999 Association of American Medical Colleges).

- Chapter 4: "The Covenant within the Covenant: Doctors and Patients in Sirach 38:1–15." *Linacre Quarterly* 55, no. 4 (1988): 14–24.
- Chapter 8: "A Biopsychosocial-Spiritual Model for the Care of Patients at the End of Life." *The Gerontologist* 42 (suppl. 3, 2002): 24–33 (© 2002 Gerontological Society of America). Reproduced by permission of the publisher.
- Chapter 12: "Healing the Dying: Spiritual Issues in the Care of the Dying Patient." In *The Health Professional as Friend and Healer*, ed. J. Kissel and D. C. Thomasma. Washington, D.C.: Georgetown University Press, 2000, 188–97 (© 2000 Georgetown University Press).
- Chapter 13: "At Wit's End: Forgiveness, Dignity, and the Care of the Dying." *Journal of General Internal Medicine* 16 (2001): 335–38 (© 2001 Blackwell Publishing).

I also would like to thank the publishers for their kind permission to reproduce quotes from the following literary works:

- "Let Evening Come," © 2005 by the estate of Jane Kenyon. Reprinted from *Collected Poems* with the permission of Graywolf Press, St. Paul, Minnesota.
- Excerpt from "Last Days," from *Without: Poems by Donald Hall*, © 1998 by Donald Hall. Reprinted by permission of Houghton Mifflin Co. All rights reserved.
- Excerpts from *W;t*, by Margaret Edson, © 1993, 1999 by Margaret Edson. Reprinted by permission of Faber and Faber, Inc., an affiliate of Farrar, Strauss and Giroux, LLC.

Introduction

Foucault's clinic is dead.[1] It was born afflicted with multiple, fatal congenital anomalies—a monster that struck terror in the hearts of many people even as it was slowly dying. Foucault's "clinic" refers to the scientific, pathological approach to medicine that emerged between the Enlightenment and the establishment of university clinics in the nineteenth century. It became the dominant form of Western medicine and persisted as the model throughout the twentieth century. Previously, sick people went to hospitals run by monks and nuns, if they were poor; if they were rich, doctors came to see them in their houses. With the rise of the clinic, however, Foucault saw the meaning of medicine change. With its scientific foundations and empirical successes, the clinic became medicine's living laboratory. Sick people came to a place where the doctors were in control. This shift in location heralded a shift in meaning. With the advent of the autopsy and anatomical pathology, diseases were analyzed by their visible effects on inner organs. Later, pathophysiology emerged as a mode of seeing diseases invisible to the untrained eye. With the birth of the clinic, Foucault saw the fundamental norms of medicine transformed. It became a practice of power; a form of control; a scientific discourse; a form of applied engineering. This revolution in medical practice brought innumerable technological advances and improvements in health, for which the world must be grateful. Despite its intelligence and giftedness, however, Foucault's clinic harbored a fatal illness. And now it has breathed its last breath. Managed care is simply its coffin.

In truth, the clinic was nearly dead by the time Foucault gave it a name. Patients left it for dead decades ago. Now even the clinicians, the masters of the clinic, have begun to acknowledge that the corpse is stiff and cold.

Where will they go, however? To whom will the sick and their healers turn?

Some have sought refuge in the new clinic of regenerative medicine, where promises of immortality are wrought from somatic cell nuclear transfer. The wise ones, however, have recognized that regenerative medicine is nothing more than the sick progeny of Foucault's clinic, bearing the same fatal congenital afflictions, worse still in each succeeding generation. Others have run to integrative medicine, seeking immortality in chants and macrobiotic diets. This trend also will pass.

Yet the desire for a new form of medicine is real and deep. People today are not ready to give up scientific progress and all that it has to offer, but they rightly sense the need for more. Their desire is spiritual. They want a form of medicine that can heal them in body and soul.

The problem with Foucault's clinic was that it was born without a soul. Paraphrasing Foucault, Ivan Illich writes, "The French Revolution gave birth to two great myths: one, that physicians could replace the clergy; the other, that with political change society would return to a state of original health."[2] Foucault's clinic promised a form of medicine that was liberated from the trappings of religion and based on science and reason. Yet the power of science, untethered from religion's moral constraints, became the source of its corruption and death. The clinic suffocated in the unanticipated by-products of medicine practiced as a merely scientific enterprise. Patients came to feel like scientific specimens rather than human beings. Iatrogenic conditions (illnesses caused by medical practice) grew steadily more prominent with every scientific success. Some side effects have been even more social than biophysical. Children who benefit from scientific medicine and do not die at the age of five now live long enough to develop Alzheimer's disease. Scientific success in treating infertility through *in vitro* fertilization is now the leading cause of premature birth. The solutions to these problems, as proposed by Foucault's clinic in its last dying days, had been diagnostic of its affliction—more nursing homes, more neonatal intensive care units, more research. Empathy and mutual acceptance of the frailty of our common humanity had come to be considered anachronistic.

The clinic had grown morbidly obese, fattened by the false promises of a scientific practice untempered by humility and unchastened by awe. Medicine came to eschew the mystical. It became blind to the mystery *within* the person of the patient and blind to the mystery that lay *beyond* the range of its scientific gaze. Having reduced the patient to a lifeless corpse—a pathological specimen—the clinic was already participating in its own death. Then, at its apparent apogee, having reduced patients to lifeless and inanimate molecules, the clinic itself became lifeless and inanimate. That is what it means to be dead.

All living bodies need souls. Otherwise, they are formless and lifeless matter. Clinics too need spirit if they are to minister to needs of the living, soulful bodies of the ill and injured human beings who enter them. The death of Foucault's clinic is an inherently unstable historical anomaly. Human beings, body and soul, still become sick and die. Other human beings still reach out to them, to help them in their bodily need, motivated by forces deep within their souls. Hence, we should not be surprised that around the globe there are signs of clinical reanimation—signs of a spiritual awakening in health care. In the twenty-first century, the clinic is being reborn.

People who are sick are looking for what Foucault's clinic failed to offer them. They seek a form of medicine that treats them as persons—a form of medicine that acknowledges what science cannot see or hear or accomplish. They want a form of medicine that does not abandon science but also does not eschew the mystical. Often, they seek this ideal in alternative forms of medical care. Most, however, want soul medicine and scientific medicine at the same time.[3] Numerous volumes about spirituality and health now fill the shelves of bookstores, catering to those needs. Physicians, nurses, and other health care professionals also are exploring the spiritual aspect of care. Some are experimenting with various means of incorporating spirituality into practice. Others are conducting empirical investigations of the effects of spirituality and religion on patients. Still others are taking stock of the spiritual lives of the people who provide patient care. Nursing schools have taught spiritual assessment for years, and courses in spirituality and health care are now becoming common in medical schools.

Yet little of this trend has been subjected to a careful examination. Not all attempts to reanimate the clinic are spiritually healthy. Critics inside and outside the healing professions are raising serious questions about what calls for reintroduction of spirituality into health care mean. Some observers seem to suggest that we should abandon centuries of scientific progress for a new form of spiritual medicine. Others reject all attempts to reintroduce spirituality into health care, fearing that it is nothing more than a disguised form of religious intolerance. Many scholars are conducting research about spirituality and health care, but without any sound theological reflection. Others reject all scientific studies of spirituality and medicine as a series of methodologically flawed investigations designed to proselytize in the pages of medical journals. Thoughtful health care professionals want to know if there is any serious, reflective basis for thinking about spirituality and health care. Above all, they want to know how it might affect their practices. This book attempts to answer some of these questions.

In part I, I explore the nature of illness and the nature of healing in an attempt to establish a solid foundation for reflection about spirituality and health care. I analyze a 2,200-year-old historical text in search of some guidance and attempt to sketch a historical dialectic of the relationship between spirituality and health care over the succeeding centuries of Western health care. I argue that the taking of oaths is the last spiritual residue left in the "official" world of mainstream contemporary medicine and suggest ways to revitalize the meaning of physicians' oaths.

In part II, I examine the recent rash of empirical studies about spirituality and patient care and attempt to separate the wheat from the chaff. I caution that there are profound limitations to the use of empirical methods in studying spirituality and health care. I propose, however, a biopsychosocial-spiritual model for health care and suggest how various kinds of empirical investigation can fit within this model. I then undertake a critique of one particularly controversial form of empirical research about spirituality and health care: randomized, controlled trials of prayer as a therapeutic intervention. Finally, I make the bold claim that health care professionals ought to regard attending to the spiritual needs of patients not just as a moral *option* but as a moral *obligation*. Contrary to much of what has appeared in the medical literature, however, I argue that empirical data have little to do with justifying that claim.

In part III, I take up some spiritual questions that arise particularly in the care of patients at the end of life. I do not intend to suggest that these issues do not occur at other clinical junctures, but the urgency with which they arise at the end of life makes it a particularly fruitful setting for thinking about these questions. In this part of the book I take up the question of praying for miracles; I flesh out some of the major spiritual themes that arise in the care of dying patients and how clinicians should deal with them; and I reflect on the play *W;t* and what playwright Margaret Edson might be able to teach health care professionals about caring for the spiritual needs of dying patients. I conclude with a personal story about the spiritual journey of one of my patients who died.

Readers should have fair warning about two general aspects of this book. First, much of this work has been drawn from talks and essays that were originally intended for a variety of audiences. Therefore the chapters vary considerably in their approach. Some are more inspirational than informational or analytical in their content and aim. Others, such as chapter 5, are philosophical and assume some background in that discipline. Some chapters mix the inspirational and the theoretical. Although this mix might be off-putting for some readers, I am convinced that, ultimately, these approaches are mutually interdependent. Genuine spirituality engages the mind as well as the heart, and complete separation between the two would undermine a significant theme of this book. Nonetheless, readers can feel free to skip any material that seems to assume too much background. For the most part, the individual chapters can stand on their own.

Second, throughout this book, I make no secret of the fact that I am a Roman Catholic and a Franciscan friar. I could not do otherwise. One can write theology in the abstract. One can write ethics in the abstract. One can write about the history of religion or even the history of spirituality in the abstract. One cannot, however, write about *spirituality* in a manner that abstracts from one's own person—one's deepest beliefs, experiences, feelings, and commitments. I trust that readers will not be offended if I profess my own conviction that the beliefs, practices, texts, rituals, and teachings of Roman Catholic Christianity express the fullness of the truth about God. This conviction does not mean that the book will be pointless for non-Catholics. It simply means that there is no point in professing any religion if one is not convinced that it is worth taking very seriously. I stake my whole spiritual being upon it. If I were not convinced that it mattered, there would be little point in the reader's taking anything that I say about spirituality very seriously.

The precise extent to which this confessional aspect of spirituality is made explicit varies considerably from chapter to chapter. Yet I hope that all of these reflections have value for a wide group of people who are interested in the broad topic of spirituality in health care—including persons of other faiths and persons of no faith. As I argue in chapter 2, I believe that health care is inherently personal and spiritual. My own belief in the doctrine of the Incarnation leads me to conclude that what is most deeply human has been touched by the Divine. If, in the course of these pages, I have pointed to that deeply human core, then I have done all I set out to do—for it is only from that core that the clinic can be reborn.

Notes

1. Michel Foucault, *The Birth of the Clinic: An Archeology of Medical Perception*, trans. A. M. Sheridan Smith (New York: Vintage, 1994). See translator's note (p. vii) for Foucault's use of the word "clinic" as a somewhat technical term.

2. Ivan Illich, *Medical Nemesis: The Expropriation of Health* (New York: Bantam Books, 1976), 151. This assertion paraphrases the discussion in Foucault, *Birth of the Clinic*, 32–33. Foucault describes an idea he attributes to the ideology of the French Revolution that medicine "would be close to the old spiritual vocation of the Church, of which it would be a sort of lay carbon copy" (32).

3. D. M. Eisenberg, R. C. Kessler, M. I. Van Rompay, T. J. Kaptchuk, S. A. Wilkey, S. Appel, and R. B. Davis, "Perceptions about Complementary Therapies Relative to Conventional Therapies among Adults Who Use Both: Results from a National Survey," *Annals of Internal Medicine* 135 (2001): 344–51.

Part I

Rebirth in the Clinic

The incorporation of spirituality into health care requires a theoretical foundation. Such a foundation serves several critical functions. To establish spirituality as the fecund ground for the rebirth of the clinic, one must have a sustainable source. To judge the moral limits and moral requirements for incorporating spirituality into practice, one must have a framework for making the necessary moral assessments. To avoid the pitfalls of charlatanism, one must have criteria by which to judge the authenticity of any proposal for incorporating spirituality into health care. The aim of part I of this book is to provide such a theoretical foundation.

The first three chapters are very general. They set forth the scope of the spiritual in health care. Chapter 4 sets forth how the ancient Jewish wisdom literature tackled the question. Chapter 5 provides my own theoretical foundation. Chapter 6 describes the role that oath-taking might play in the spiritual rebirth of the clinic.

Many good things have been happening in the field of spirituality and health care. Several initiatives, however, have suffered from a lack of focus. I start by examining the spirituality and health care movement through a theoretical lens, beginning with a look at the most basic aspects of spiritual experience in the clinic and constructing a framework for understanding what has already happened and what needs to happen next.

$\sim\!\!\mathbb{O}$ 1

Why Surgeons Must Be Very Careful

More than 150 years ago Emily Dickinson wrote a poem that succinctly illuminates many of the spiritual aspects of practicing the healing arts.[1] She lived and wrote when the modern scientific clinic was just coming into its own. She had a keen sense of diagnosis; she understood immediately what ailed the clinic. She wrote, in her typically pithy style:

> Surgeons must be very careful
> When they take the knife!
> Underneath their fine incisions
> Stirs the Culprit—*Life!*

Whenever this poem creeps into the contemporary medical literature, as it sometimes does, it usually is an epigraph at the beginning of an article that emphasizes the importance of good surgical technique. These days, however, this poem might sound more like a stern warning from a risk manager or advice from a newspaper reporter, a judge, a politician, or perhaps an angry patient—or someone else who distrusts physicians and surgeons and is skeptical about their competence, sincerity, or commitment to patient welfare. Be careful, doc!

We should be more careful readers, however, because Dickinson was a very careful poet. She chose each of her words very carefully to be richly suggestive and highly evocative. Moreover, her insights are important for all health care professionals—not just surgeons.

3

Begin with the word *take*. This word evokes the power one has as a physician, surgeon, or nurse—a power to heal or to harm, even to kill. A clinician's knowledge, as Bacon observed, also is power. Clinicians wield knowledge over their patients, who are at the mercy of that knowledge. Like all power, the power clinicians hold can be used for good or evil—and mostly, if we are honest, for some admixture of both.

The word *take* also suggests the verb phrase *take up*, and this interpretation makes the word more interesting. Medicine is a craft (in Greek, *techne*). One takes up the medical craft, in some ways, just as one says that someone has taken up gardening or pottery. Physicians, however, do not make anything in their craft. The product of their craft is not something of their own making, like a piece of clothing or furniture or a utensil. The patient is given to a physician, and the physician gives the patient back to herself and to her family. Although medicine is a genuine craft, it is, one must admit, a funny sort of craft.

Consider also Dickinson's use of the word *fine*. This word suggests the precision of the physician's work. Technical specialties and subspecialties—such as head and neck surgery, neurosurgery, and invasive cardiology—are especially precise crafts, dealing with the delicate sense organs and the myriad fragile nerves and vessels that traverse the body. Yet even a general internist, pediatrician, or nurse must be precise. An error of a decimal point in dosing can mean the difference between cure and death.

Yet the word *fine* also evokes a sense of the beauty of what clinicians do. Surgery can restore the beauty of a face deformed by genetic processes gone awry or palliate the distortions of injury or cancer. Medication can erase the disfigurement wrought by diseases such as Kaposi's sarcoma or leprosy. Often there is a beauty to the intervention itself—an aesthetic of the craft. Surgical incisions can have their own beauty, running down the natural folds of the neck or the linea alba so that no one who looks at the patient in a few years will discern that a surgeon was ever there. Even case presentations have a beauty—at least if they are done well. Crispness, clarity, brevity, vitality, and precision characterize a good presentation of a case. There is a genuine aesthetics of case presentations.

Dickinson's poem itself has all the qualities of a good case presentation. Yet perhaps it is better to say that a good case presentation is like one of Dickinson's poems. In each art form, every word counts. So we may also read her "fine incisions" as a reminder that all clinicians must be incisive. A pediatrician must know how to sense when something is askew in a parent's reaction to a child's fractured bone. An internist must recognize those moments when therapy is required even in the absence of a precise diagnosis. A surgeon must make incisions, not just cuts. The difference between an incision and a cut must be part of the surgeon's character. Yet the best surgeons are always conscious as they dissect a path through tissue planes and remove diseased nodes that they are opening up more than flesh. Surgeons also expose the *persons* of their patients in a psychosocial and even a spiritual sense. All good clinicians are as incisive about persons as they are about malignancies.

Dickinson therefore seems to be urging the clinician to get "underneath" what he or she is doing—not just underneath the skin (in the anatomical-pathological sense of Foucault's clinic) but underneath the experience that the physician shares with the patient. One might read Dickinson as imploring physicians (or, more broadly, anyone who applies technology to human beings) to resist the urge to be callous or superficial or to trivialize what they do. Such reactions might appear to help in the short term but will return to haunt the practitioner in the long term.

The work of all health care professionals is fraught with deeper meaning than they often realize. Clinicians and pathologists alike often experience the patient in frozen sections—thin slices of flesh, frozen in time. Dickinson seems to urge all health care professionals to remember that the moment of the clinical encounter is also but a frozen section: a thin slice of the patient, frozen in time, revealing nothing about the hopes and fears and loves and sorrows the patient brings to the encounter at levels far deeper than any surgeon can ever reach with any knife, deeper than any medical imaging technique can ever bring to light.

This, then, is what "stirs" beneath the surgeon's knife. Even when a patient is sedated, paralyzed, and ventilated, the mystery of a person stirs dynamically at the tips of the surgeon's fingers. It is the profound mystery of the person that stirs—not just blood, but Life.

Life is what stirs—in all its richness, power, and mystery. It is Life that health care professionals serve. Clinicians understand this perspective best when they come to understand the way their own lives are deeply connected with the lives of their patients. Yet life in the modern clinic can make this concept difficult to comprehend. Particularly in delivering highly technical medical care—in the endoscopy suite, in the cardiac catheterization laboratory, in the surgical theater—one may be so bound up with the patient that one scarcely notices anything more than the concentration, tension, and exactitude of one's work. Well, one should be fixed on the technical, clinical moment, as such, while it is unfolding. Yet this necessary focus does not excuse any health care professional from the duty to reflect on what he or she actually does, day in and day out. All health care professionals are at the service of Life. It stirs at the bottom of the surgical field. It courses through the physician's veins as surely as it flows through those of the patient.

Dickinson does not suggest that one should worship this Life. She is not a vitalist. Her poem is not a call to never cease treatment, nor is she delivering a moral mandate to maintain the ventilator even if the patient is brain dead. She calls modern practitioners to an attitude that Albert Schweitzer once called "reverence for life."[2] This attitude is one of awe and respect. It commands action to heal and preserve Life—but true reverence for Life is tempered by realism. One should not desecrate Life for the sake of preserving mitochondrial oxidative phosphorylation.

Hence, Dickinson observes that Life is a culprit—and she is right. One might take up the knife or the syringe and think one wields its power, but Life steals that power back. Life ought to make one humble and steal away one's arrogance. Physicians and surgeons ought to grasp (as they are in turn grasped by) the paradox of this Life. Life itself brings both illness and health to everyone. Life by its very nature is finite: Every patient will die one day, and surgery, medicine, and nursing ultimately are powerless to stop it.

Life holds within it the seeds of death—apoptosis. Life is the context of illness. If there were no Life, there could be no illness. Life is defined over and against Death—the ultimate expression of our finitude. Illness is the mark of the finitude of life. Things go wrong for living things. That is their nature. Illness arises because living things (all living things, including physicians) are marked by mistakes—biochemically, physiologically, socially, intellectually, morally, and spiritually.

Thus, like Life itself, the medical craft is marked by its finitude. Everyone makes mistakes. This is why clinicians feel so much more hurt than angry when their mistakes become the headlines of bad press and the source of lawsuits. Imperfection marks the healing crafts. Yet in the face of the inevitability of every patient's ultimate dissolution, and with the full knowledge of their own metaphysically certain insufficiency for the task, health care professionals serve Life.

Health care professionals sometimes forget that Life itself is the healer, not them. Where there is any success, the craft only contributes to the healing that Life itself offers. Life is the source of all illness and the source of all healing. Health care professionals help, but they are not the source of healing. No matter how sophisticated surgery may be, it would not even be possible if the body did not heal itself.

So, Life is a culprit. Life gives, and Life takes away. Life deals out both healing and sickness. Life deals out birth and death. Life gives health care professionals the power to heal and snatches it away when they become too possessive.

Perhaps the reader might be thinking that this discussion is all too abstract—the irrelevant musings of an internist with a PhD in philosophy who happens to be a Franciscan friar and thinks he can interpret poems. This notion became very real for me in 2003, however. In April of that year my uncle was diagnosed with squamous cell carcinoma of the tongue. In May he was admitted to my hospital, where he underwent partial glossectomy and radical lymph node dissection, followed by radiation therapy.

My uncle asked all the questions such patients ask. "What does this mean?" First, "Is it serious?" Later, "What are my chances?" "How did this happen?" "Should I blame the dentist who kept telling me for six months that the sore on my tongue was due to ill-fitting dentures?"

"Was it my smoking and drinking? But doc, I've been sober for 25 years, and I quit smoking 30 years ago."

I wondered whether my uncle's experience brought up memories of his son, who had died at the age of five of acute lymphoblastic leukemia. Would he blame God again? Would he start drinking again? His wife said simply, "He don't talk about things like that."

Life *is* a culprit. Life gives, and Life takes away.

I helped my uncle navigate the overly bureaucratic U.S. health care system. I ran down a radiologist friend in the hallway just to print out a copy of my uncle's CT scan for him to bring to his PET scan, scheduled for the following day. Apparently a hospital clerk had informed my uncle that the hospital was out of film and would not be able to supply the copy of the CT scan that the insurance company and clerks at the PET scan office had said would be necessary for him to have his PET scan. The PET scan was scheduled for the following morning. I didn't share with my uncle that the reason our hospital was out of film was that the vicissitudes of market medicine had rendered the hospital nearly bankrupt, so it couldn't pay its bills, leading the X-ray film company to refuse to deliver us any more film on credit. I begged and pleaded, and the radiologist and I found some film not already designated for emergencies. We printed a copy of the CT scan for my uncle and thereby avoided a tense and confusing situation for him.

Later that night, however, my uncle called me in a panic. The PET scan center now said they were canceling his scheduled PET scan because the proper managed care authorization form had not been filled out. I called his surgeon, who promptly filled it out and faxed it to the billing clerk at the for-profit, freestanding PET scan center. Stage two of my uncle's potential bureaucratic nightmare had been averted. I wondered, however, what happens to patients who don't have a nephew on the medical staff?

I think my uncle and his wife and daughters and his surgeon lived an experience that makes them understand the importance of what Emily Dickinson had to say. Their story makes the poem real.

This story brings me back to the word *careful*. Why is that word so important in Dickinson's poem? It certainly does not mean a posture of medico-legal risk management—being careful to cover one's behind. Nor does it mean mere technical precision.

Dickinson urges us, as health care professionals, to be full of care. Care has many meanings that are relevant to the work of a clinician. German philosopher Hans-Georg Gadamer has written some things in his book, *The Enigma of Health*, that can help us understand better what Dickinson means.[3]

In part, care means solicitude. Gadamer reminds us that a careful clinician is solicitous toward the patient.[4]

Care also means that the patient most often is full of cares—*Sorgen* in German; we also render that meaning of *cares* as *worries* or *anxieties* in English. A careful clinician is attentive to the cares of the patient.[5]

Gadamer also explores how the German word for treatment, *Behandlung*, suggests careful handling of the patient. Physicians and surgeons begin with palpation—touching their patients in intimate ways. Gadamer describes palpation as, "carefully and responsively feeling the patient's body so as to detect strains and tensions which can perhaps help to confirm or correct the patient's own subjective localization, that is, the patient's experience of pain."[6]

How can one cultivate such care? In the *Phaedrus*, Plato makes three puzzling claims, one after the other: that rhetoric should be considered the same as medicine, that it is not possible to understand the soul without considering it as a whole, and that—if we are to believe Hippocrates the Asclepiad—we cannot begin to understand the body without considering the whole.[7] Gadamer's interpretation of what Plato is saying can be summarized as follows: that just as philosophy only emerges out of dialogue, the same is true of medicine, and that just as philosophy must be holistic, so must medicine.[8]

In other words, Plato suggests that real medicine must be soul medicine. One cannot know the whole patient merely through science. The medical act emerges through a dialogue with the patient. Even the examination of the patient; one's careful handling of the patient; one's touching without words, is a dialogue. One does not merely touch the carotid artery as an object. One touches the patient's soul. Therefore, one must be very, very careful.

Since the time of the ancient Greeks, illness has been understood as a disturbance in equilibrium. All attempts to heal are always a counterforce. Gadamer reminds us, however, that there is always a threat, therefore, of doing too much.[9]

A story illustrates this point. Dr. John Conley was a famous head and neck surgeon who practiced many years at my hospital, St. Vincent's Hospital in New York City. Conley is considered one of the founders of the field of head and neck surgery, transforming it far beyond "ear, nose, and throat" medicine. As is often the case with pioneering figures, he also was a very colorful character. I have been told by one of his former residents that in the middle of very difficult and complex cancer operations he often would stop what he was doing, put down the instruments, and with a characteristically dramatic flair, begin to ask questions.

"What's that?" he would ask, pointing at something in the surgical field.

A resident would answer, with quivering lips, "The jugular vein."

"What's that?" he would ask again, pointing elsewhere. A knock-kneed medical student would say, "It looks like more tumor."

Then Conley would ask, "Are you sure?" The resident would save the medical student from any possible embarrassment by answering, "Yes."

"And what might happen to this human being before us if we attempt to remove this tumor?" No one would answer.

"Should we proceed?" No one would answer.

Then he would simply say to the nurse, "Scalpel."

Conley was trying to teach the residents and students assembled in his operating room how to be careful surgeons. He was Socratic and dialogical with his students as well as with his patients. His comments concerned technique, certainly. The point he was making, however, was about far more than technique. It was about human beings and human Life. He demonstrated, in dramatic gesture, that before Life, the careful surgeon must give pause. Gadamer writes that when a medical intervention goes wrong, "it would not be because physical force or power was lacking or too little was exerted, but rather because there was actually too much force in play. But when the act works, suddenly everything seems to happen spontaneously, lightly and effortlessly. . . . Genuine success is accomplished in medical practice at just that point where intervention is rendered superfluous and dispensable. All medical efforts at healing are already conceived from the outset in light of the fact that the doctor's contribution consummates itself by disappearing as soon as the equilibrium of health is restored."[10]

Life gives the physician the power to heal and then takes it back again. That is what Conley's little operating room drama was about. Although not all clinicians have his dramatic flair, at some point—at least symbolically—each clinician should put down the knife he or she has taken up and revere the mystery he or she is privileged to serve.

Gadamer points out, in fact, that the word *therapy* comes from the Greek *therapeia*, which means service.[11] Being a careful clinician means seeing oneself as the patient's servant, not as the patient's lord and master.

Several years ago, a young woman named Helen Yoo Bowne took the knife to my uncle Denis. She is a careful surgeon. She did not take up the knife as an implement of power. Her incisions were very fine. She understood the mystery that lay beneath the plane of all possible dissection. I was very touched by the way she took the time, after eight hours of surgery, to speak with his wife and daughters while her patient was being taken to the recovery room. She engaged them in respectful dialogue. She answered their questions in clear and simple language. She communicated compassion and concern. She broke with hospital protocol to allow them to visit him in the recovery room so they could finally go home rather than waiting until he was out of recovery and in a bed. The first thing he remembered after waking up in the recovery room was the voice of his wife. A careful surgeon, practicing soul medicine, gave him that gift.

These days, in the face of all the troubles (cares, if you will) that beset the health care professions, one hears more and more discussion of physician work stoppages, unionization, and media campaigns to restore respect. I confess to being skeptical about these approaches. Health care professionals often are unjustly beleaguered, but they also need to earn back patients' respect and trust. There is no better way of doing so than by concentrating on the basics, becoming again who we always have known we should be—physicians, surgeons, nurses, and others who are full of care; humble, sincere, compassionate, and competent. The Culprit that stirs beneath the fine incisions we make in our patients stirs deep beneath the wounds in our own collective psyche. We must never forget that.

Notes

1. Emily Dickinson, number 156, in *The Poems of Emily Dickinson*, Variorum ed., vol. 1, ed. R. W. Franklin (Cambridge, Mass.: Belknap Press of Harvard University Press, 1998), 194. This poem is number 108 in the Johnson edition.

2. Albert Schweitzer, *Out of My Life and Thought: An Autobiography*, trans. Antje Bultmann Lemke (Baltimore: Johns Hopkins University Press, 1998), 155–59.

3. Hans-Georg Gadamer, *The Enigma of Health: The Art of Healing in a Scientific Age*, trans. Jason Gaiger and Nicholas Walker (Stanford, Calif.: Stanford University Press, 1996).

4. Ibid., 157.

5. Ibid., 159.

6. Ibid., 108.

7. Plato, *Phaedrus* 270–71, trans. W. C. Hemhold and W. G. Rabinowitz (Indianapolis: Bobbs-Merrill, Library of the Liberal Arts, 1956), 60–64.

8. Gadamer, *Enigma of Health*, 131–32.

9. Ibid., 114.

10. Ibid., 37.

11. Ibid., 128.

~~ 2

Is Health Care a Spiritual Practice?

Is health care a spiritual practice? Although this question is central to this book, it must seem odd to most people in the Western world today. Most would agree that health care is the most delicate and intricate form of applied science. Most also probably would agree that what is not science in health care could be called art—the making of particular judgments about particular patients. Many would agree that there is a poetic beauty to some aspects of the practice of this art, as well as a need for a deeper sense of care and compassion in medicine. Yet the question remains: Are medicine, nursing, dentistry, psychology, and the other healing professions really spiritual practices? What would the skeptic say?

"Not since the Middle Ages! The era of witchcraft is thankfully behind us. The era of molecular medicine is dawning." If anything, many clinicians might believe that chaplains could be of some limited use to some patients, helping them cope with illness. This spiritual element would be adjunctive, however. It would not be "*real* health care."

What has spirituality to do with health care, or health care with spirituality?

Spirituality and Religion

The answer may first depend on what one means by spirituality. Many people equate spirituality with religion. Yet although these words are conceptually related, they are not synonymous.[1]

13

Religious traditions are deeply related at the spiritual level. Religious traditions sometimes even trade spiritual practices back and forth. For instance, prayer beads were common to Hindu, Buddhist, and Islamic practice, and some religious historians have hypothesized that Franciscan missionaries to the Middle East brought the idea back with them to medieval Europe, providing a tallying method for the developing practice of recited Marian prayers that eventually became known as the rosary.[2]

Hence, in a sense illustrated by this observation, spirituality is a much broader term than religion. One's spirituality may be defined simply as the characteristics and qualities of one's relationship with the transcendent. It includes attitudes, habits, and practices in relation to the idea of the transcendent. Thus, everyone may be said to have a spirituality. Many people call the transcendent "God." One also may live in relationship with the transcendent and refuse to personalize it or call it "God." Even if one explicitly rejects the existence of the transcendent, one has a relationship with it—at least by way of rejecting it. By this broad definition, even an atheist has a spirituality because an atheist must search for personal meaning and value in light of his or her rejection of the possibility of a transcendent source of personal meaning and value.

By contrast, a religion is a specific set of beliefs about the transcendent, held in common by a community of persons, usually in association with a particular language used to describe spiritual experiences and a communal sharing of key beliefs, along with particular associated practices, texts, rituals, and teachings. In a religion people share some basic, overarching assumptions about the transcendent. Not everyone has a religion.

It has become increasingly common in the United States for people to describe themselves as "spiritual but not religious."[3] By the definitions I have offered, this description is not oxymoronic or otherwise logically impossible. Whether being "spiritual but not religious" is personally, socially, and theologically sustainable is another matter. It cannot be dismissed out of hand, however. Moreover, this position is becoming more prevalent.

One contemporary consequence of the fact that religions have so much in common at the level of spiritual practice has been the emergence (particularly among people who are "spiritual but not religious") of multiple personal, syncretistic styles of spiritual practice. People in the postindustrial Western world increasingly eschew organized religion, yet they borrow spiritual teachings from multiple traditions to create an individualized set of spiritual practices. Although I write from a particular religious tradition, I hope such readers will not be deterred. For many readers, what I hold to be the fullness of spiritual truth may be merely one voice among many. As I state in the Introduction, however, the fact that one does not share my faith should not be an impediment to reading this book.

Religious traditions do have a great deal to offer to doctors, nurses, dentists, and psychologists, as well as their patients. People who set out on a spiritual quest and already have a religion are very fortunate in one sense. They already have a language, texts, a community, and a set of practices with which to express their experiences of the transcendent and in which to cultivate their spiritual lives. Inventing all this for oneself is immensely difficult. The eclectic approach does not provide a spiritual community. It distances itself from any and all particular traditions. Echoing Wittgenstein's comments regarding the impossibility of private language, I would even contend that the eclectic approach does not constitute an alternative form of religion.[4] There is no such thing as a private religion. There can be private spirituality, but not private religion. Furthermore, private, religionless spirituality will simply always be harder to live than religious spirituality.

I am fully persuaded, however, that if a Christian speaks out of the fullness of Christian conviction, and a Buddhist speaks out of the fullness of Buddhist conviction, and an atheist speaks out of the fullness of atheist conviction, deep spiritual resonances will occur and each can learn enormously from the others. Although in one sense spirituality is broader than religion, in another sense spirituality ultimately is more specific than religion. Within every religion there are groups of people who share the key beliefs of the religion and remain part of the community of believers, yet have slightly different ways of praying, as well as other slightly different ways of living out their relationships with the transcendent. Thus, within the broad Catholic Church there are charismatics and traditionalists; Dominicans, Jesuits, Benedictines, and Franciscans; people who pray the rosary and people who practice centering prayer—all distinct spiritualities within one religion.

Ultimately, because every human personality is unique, every human relationship with the transcendent also is unique. Spirituality therefore is ultimately personal. Only persons can apprehend, question, and live lives that engage the transcendent. Hence, this book is addressed to *persons*.

Spirituality and Health Care Practice

At this point the reader may ask, legitimately, what does any of this have to do with health care practice? One reply comes from Abraham Heschel, the twentieth-century Jewish philosopher and theologian. Heschel once said in an address to the American Medical Association, "To heal a person, one must first be a person."[5] This understanding is the first step in building a spirituality for health care.

Etymologically, to heal means to make whole. If health care professionals are committed to healing patients as whole persons, they must understand not only what disease and injury do to patients' bodies but also what disease and injury do to them as embodied spiritual persons grappling with transcendent questions.

In the midst of all that is being written and said these days about spirituality and health care, surprisingly little has been discussed about the spiritual lives of physicians and nurses. As Heschel reminds us, if health care professionals are to heal patients as whole persons, they themselves must seriously engage the transcendent questions that only persons can ask. If health care professionals are to be true healers, they must rediscover what it means for health care to be a spiritual practice.

The relationship between health care and spirituality has become problematic in the twenty-first century as it never was in earlier eras— and is not for many non-Western cultures today. A simple story illustrates this point. A Roman Catholic couple went to Easter mass on a Canadian reservation where a native North American bishop was presiding in his tribal language. The couple, both physicians, were the only white people in the church. The bishop's sermon was lengthy. As he preached, every once in a while he turned to the couple, acknowledging his awareness that they understood nothing of what he was saying. At the end of a thirty-minute sermon, he turned to the guests and welcomed them in broken English on behalf of his congregation. He offered to summarize his sermon. He paused for a moment and then said simply, "This Jesus. *Strong* medicine."

Efficacious, scientific Western medicine also is strong, but is it strong enough? Western health care works, and very few people want to give up antibiotics or neurosurgery in favor of crystals. Is it not possible, however, to practice excellent scientific medicine, nursing, dentistry, psychology, and other health professions and still be aware of the spiritual dimension of the work and responsive to the spiritual needs of patients?

Illness is a spiritual event. Illness grasps persons by the soul as well as by the body and disturbs both. Illness ineluctably raises troubling questions of a transcendent nature—questions about meaning, value, and relationship. These questions are spiritual. How health care professionals answer these questions for themselves will affect the way they help their patients struggle with these questions.

We know so little about the ways in which we touch the lives of our patients—or about the ways in which we fail them. Some time ago, for example, I found myself in a discussion with a nurse about the role of touch in relation to health care and spirituality. She had misinterpreted something I had said during a lecture, and to demonstrate, somewhat defensively, that I really did believe in touching patients, I asked if she would mind if I showed her how I generally auscultate the lungs, placing my right hand on the patient's right shoulder. I demonstrated: "Like so." She then responded, "Oh. Do you know what that does to patients? What it communicates?" Even more defensive and stunned, I said, "No." She then asked permission to demonstrate on me. She said, "You could touch people like this," and she leaned a bit on my shoulder to balance herself in a perfunctory manner. "But that's not what you do. Here's what you do." Then she touched my shoulder in such an amazing way that it seemed at the same time as if she were not touching me; in a manner that communicated confidence and compassion at once; in a way that signified respect and connection at once. It felt as if a static charge hovered between her hand and my shoulder. Yet she really was touching me, and there was no space between us. "Is that really what I do?" I asked. "I guess so," she said. "That's what you did when you demonstrated for me."

"Wow," I thought. "Strong medicine."

From my perspective, the transcendent, healing presence of the divine can be found in the interstices of daily practice—in the infinite space that subsists between our hands and the bodies of the patients we touch. Too few of us bother to reflect on it or talk to each other about it. The transcendent, healing presence of the divine is to be found not only in explicitly religious conversation with patients who are dying but in countless moments in the office or the hospital in which we communicate meaning and value to our patients and relate to them as persons. A drug such as adriamycin doesn't necessarily get in the way of understanding the clinical encounter as a spiritual experience, although it can. If we use a drug incompetently, we violate the trust the patient has placed in us—a trust that transcends the relationship between patient and professional and transcends adriamycin. To betray that trust is to deny the spirit.

Adriamycin also can get in the way of the spirit if we somehow come to believe the falsehood that the patient's story (or our own story) begins and ends in adriamycin. There are no transcendent pharmaceutical agents. There are always transcendent questions, however—about meaning, value, and relationship. Spirituality in practice begins when the doctor or nurse becomes aware that these questions arise in and through illness and injury and that they can be addressed in and through health care practice. Paul Ramsey reminds us that patients are first and foremost persons.[6] We must begin to recognize that physicians, nurses, and other health care professionals also are first and foremost persons.

The Emmaus Story

The story of Emmaus, from the Gospel of Luke (24:13–35), may be very familiar to some readers and completely new to others. The story is about two disciples of Jesus, walking down the road from Jerusalem to a town named Emmaus a few days after Jesus had been crucified and buried, their hearts heavy with a sense of profound loss. As the story develops, Jesus comes up to them on the road and begins to walk with them and engage them in conversation. The story says that they did not recognize him at first. Hours later, however, when they stop at an inn along the road and share supper, they suddenly recognize him, whereupon he vanishes from their sight.

A rarely asked question about this story is this: What prevented the disciples from recognizing Jesus? It seems so strange. He was their friend, and they didn't recognize him. What could have prevented them from recognizing him?

A bit of speculation about this question is instructive. Perhaps the disciples were just a little too self-absorbed. Perhaps they were too busy complaining that the glory days were gone. Perhaps they just had too little faith to believe that it was possible for Jesus to appear to them. Perhaps they were too busy telling their story to listen to his.

Perhaps it was just grief—a deep sense of the loss of one they had loved and for whom they had cared. Perhaps it was a sense of failure—that they were powerless to keep him from dying.

The disciples only recognized Jesus later, when they took time to reflect on what was happening in their lives. When they did, they said, "Were our hearts not burning within us when he spoke to us on the way?"

Perhaps health care professionals, like the disciples on the way to Emmaus, simply have been prevented from seeing.

I invite the reader to bring to mind some morning in practice. Whenever it may have been, call it "yesterday." Allow me to share one of my yesterdays.

Yesterday morning on rounds, I saw a seventy-year-old veteran with altered mental status and a recurrent parotid cancer. He lives alone. His appearance was disheveled. He was confused and tearful. The 10 centimeter incision was weeping pus, and it smelled. He had a new 3 centimeter mass in front of his ear.

I also saw a forty-seven-year-old alcoholic grandmother with AIDS who looked at least sixty-seven. She had *Pneumocystis carinii* pneumonia, thrush, and oral and genital herpes. Yet there was a remarkable, quiet kindness and gratitude in her eyes. I can still see it.

I also saw a thirty-one-year-old man with AIDS and fulminant pulmonary Kaposi's sarcoma. He was on a respirator. His sister was the only member of the family who knew he had AIDS. He was absolutely terrified. The chemotherapy began within an hour after the bronchoscopy. I left the room doubting we would be able to save him, no matter how heroic our efforts.

I also saw a man who had spent the past eleven months in a coma, identified simply as "unknown Hispanic male." He had been hit by a car while trying to cross New York's FDR Drive. Remarkably, he had started to wake up. He still had a tracheostomy and was paralyzed and could not talk. But he was waking up. Painstakingly, we learned that his name is José, that he had been living in Queens before the accident, that he had no family in New York, and that his mother lives somewhere in Puerto Rico, but not in the city of San Juan. He smiled yesterday for the first time in eleven months. He's awake. He's alive. His name is José.

I saw him yesterday morning. You saw him yesterday on your morning rounds as well. Were your hearts not burning within you? Did you not learn from him how much the Messiah had to suffer before entering into his glory? Did he not open up the scriptures for you? It happened just yesterday. Or were your eyes prevented from recognizing him?

Barriers to Spirituality in Health Care

Multiple barriers stand in the way of this "repersonalization" of health care—this rebirth of health care as a spiritual enterprise. The present economic reconstruction of health care surely is one of these barriers.

Health care has been reconceptualized to be like any other industry; the chief virtue in health care no longer is compassion, empathy, or fidelity to trust. The chief virtue of industry is efficiency. Working in a system in which all parts are considered interchangeable and any patient can see any physician or nurse about any problem in any place at any time, believing that questions about relationships have transcendent meaning becomes more difficult.

Working in a system in which financial incentives have been reconfigured to make physician and patient economic rivals, it is hard for either patients or physicians to feel that their value constitutes true dignity—the value that has no price and belongs only to persons.[7] This is the value of those created in the image and likeness of God.

Working in a system in which patient visits have been reduced to seven minutes, it becomes almost unimaginable that questions of meaning can be addressed. Yet these neglected questions of meaning constitute the spiritual in health care.

The spirituality of medical practice therefore must begin with frank acknowledgment of how much health care professionals are suffering today. Many doctors, nurses, and other health care professionals now long to be able to give the spiritual questions of practice their due. Too many, however, find their efforts thwarted by demands to shorten the time they spend with patients, to fill out more forms, to refer patients to specialists they have never met, and to treat patients with formulary-approved drugs they have never used before. This spiritual suffering has two sources. Scientific reductionism has threatened the spiritual aspects of medical practice from within, by denying the existence of the transcendent. The industrialization of health care now threatens the spiritual aspects of medical practice from without, denying the importance of the spiritual.

Yet no amount of economic transformation can alter the fundamental meaning and value of health care, nor can it ever eradicate the interpersonal nature of the healing relationship that begins when one person feels ill and another, highly skilled and socially authorized, asks, "How can I help you?" The spirituality of medical practice at the dawn of the twenty-first century in the United States therefore demands great virtue—courage, hope, perseverance, and creative fidelity.[8] It certainly is not easy to be a health care professional today. When all is said and done, however, we know that we still touch patients in remarkable ways. The spiritual meaning of health care will outlast all mergers, all managed care organizations, all Medicare and Medicaid cutbacks, all bogus accusations of fraud and abuse, all malpractice suits, all direct-to-consumer advertising for drugs, and all manner of profiteering at the expense of patients. If spirituality is real, it is real for times of trial as well as times of triumph. Money can't buy spirituality—and money can't make it go away.

Cultivating a Spiritual Practice

How might one cultivate a spiritual sensibility in health care that will be credible in the twenty-first century? First, if one takes one's own religion seriously, one should begin to deepen one's own spiritual life within that religion. Religion makes grappling with spiritual questions easier, providing a community of faith and support and a ready-made language with which to describe spiritual struggles and joys. Religion can give a doctor or nurse practices and texts that can be starting points for a deeper exploration of the spiritual life.

Patients struggle with all the big questions: What is the meaning of my illness? Why must I suffer? Is there anything about me that is valuable now that I am no longer "productive"? What is broken in my relationships that I somehow feel called to fix now that my body is broken? Can my doctor possibly understand what I am really going through? A doctor or nurse who has begun to explore these questions in his or her own life will be better prepared to help patients struggle with these questions. Christianity and the other major religious traditions do not give pat answers to these questions that are so fundamental to the human condition. Doctors and nurses who have taken these questions seriously will not trivialize or dismiss the questions of their patients or dispense spiritual bromides to those who struggle with the mysteries of being human in the face of illness and death.

Second, one can find fellow health care professionals with whom to engage these questions. What is the meaning of health care? What is its value? What are right and good healing relationships about? These questions are spiritual. They arise ineluctably for believers and nonbelievers—for all health care professionals who take both being practitioners and persons seriously. These questions are not often discussed in the doctor's dining room. Silence can constitute its own conspiracy, however. We can learn from our patients and from each other. How do we deal with our fallibility? With the deaths of our patients? Can we move beyond kvetching about the pressures we now face? Can we see our work as service? Do we ever pray for our patients? Or pray about ourselves as healers? Have we ever experienced the transcendent in our work? Can such peak experiences sustain us? If we do not talk about these issues, we might begin to doubt the fundamental soundness of our own spiritual struggles.

To heal a person, one must first be a person. We are all spiritual beings. Health care is a spiritual discipline.

Notes

1. Daniel P. Sulmasy, *The Healer's Calling: A Spirituality for Physicians and Other Health Care Professionals* (New York, Paulist Press, 1997), 10–12.

2. Anne Winston-Allen, *Stories of the Rose: The Making of the Rosary in the Middle Ages* (University Park: University of Pennsylvania Press, 1997), 13–15.

3. See, for instance, Don Lattin, "Living the Religious Life of None: Growing Numbers Shed Organized Church for Loose Spiritual Sensibility," *San Francisco Chronicle*, December 4, 2003, A1; Barry A. Kosmin and Egon Mayer, "American Religious Identification Survey 2001"; available at http://www.gc.cuny.edu/faculty/research_studies/aris.pdf.

4. Ludwig Wittgenstein, *Philosophical Investigations* (§§ 244–78), trans. G. E. M. Anscombe (Oxford: Blackwell, 1968), 89–96.

5. Abraham J. Heschel, *The Insecurity of Freedom* (New York: Noonday Press/Farrar, Strauss, Giroux, 1966), 24–38.

6. Paul Ramsey, *The Patient as Person* (New Haven, Conn.: Yale University Press, 1970).

7. Immanuel Kant, *Grounding for the Metaphysics of Morals* (Ak 435), trans. James W. Ellington (Indianapolis: Hackett, 1981), 40–41.

8. Gabriel Marcel, *Creative Fidelity* (New York: Crossroad, 1982).

3

Dignity, Vulnerability, and the Personhood of the Patient

Several years ago some of the friars of my province decided that they wanted to use an old friary, located in a parish in northern New Jersey, to start an AIDS hospice. We had retained the friary but had given up the parish to the diocese years before. This decision came in the days before protease inhibitors, when mortality from HIV infection was still high in the United States. Vociferous opposition arose from the residents of that New Jersey town as soon as they heard of the friars' plans. Local political authorities, initially supportive, began to vacillate.

The Franciscan Provincial administration and the friars involved decided to confront this opposition head on, so the friars asked the pastor for permission to use his church basement for a "town hall" meeting to answer questions from parishioners. I was asked to take the train up from Washington, D.C., where I lived at the time, to answer medical and ethical questions.

The first sign that things would not go very well was that the pastor did not show up. We had to scramble to find a custodian to open the basement to the church. Once we were assembled, the friar in charge of the project began the meeting by relating how the idea to use the old friary as an AIDS hospice had evolved. He then invited me to stand up to answer medical and ethical questions. What ensued went far beyond "NIMBY" ("Not In My Back Yard"). It even went far beyond "BANANA"

("Build Absolutely Nothing Anywhere Near Anybody"). I witnessed pure, unadulterated hatred. First someone shouted out that no questions about medicine or ethics were relevant, so I should sit down. Then, one after another, parishioners took to the microphone and railed on in the most angry and hostile terms imaginable about declining property values; about the perverts who would prey on their children in the schoolyard across the street; and about how children would contract HIV from dirty needles. I saw the faces of what otherwise seemed like loving grandmothers snarling with such hostile expressions that I thought I was staring at Satan himself. The final straw for me, however, came when a woman stood up, identified herself as an emergency room nurse, and shouted, "I pick scum like this up off the streets of Newark every night. I don't want none of 'em in my neighborhood."

Distraught after my return to Washington, I recounted the story to an older and wiser friar with whom I lived. He remarked, "I can see that the Gospel has sunk deep roots in New Jersey."

I begin with such a negative story because I think it helps to illustrate what is at stake in the themes I discuss in this chapter. What must be preserved and yet is always in danger of being lost in health care is the complex nexus between dignity, vulnerability, and the personhood of the patient.

Dignity: The History of an Idea

The word *dignity* seems very important in contemporary discussions of health care. One hears about the dignity of the patient and about death with dignity on a frequent basis. I begin my reflections with a historical account of this word, going a long way back in time. Before this brief flight into intellectual history, however, several caveats are appropriate.

First, the rudiments of a concept of the dignity of the human person probably have been lurking in Western thought for many centuries. The point of my historical discussion is simply that the label *dignity* has not been applied consistently to that concept until relatively recently. Until it was named, there was no organized concept of human dignity.

Second, the arguments and the history I review are far more complex than I can possibly cover adequately in a brief chapter. I am trying to present a broad overview only, not a close, detailed, carefully nuanced historical, philosophical, or textual analysis. I hope that these preliminary thoughts might help to foster greater clarity about this important concept.

Scripture

To begin the historical analysis, I start with scripture. Many people, especially Catholics, might surmise that the concept of human dignity has a strong scriptural basis. In fact, however, such an assumption is incorrect. There really is no well-developed, explicit theme in scripture extolling the dignity of human life, the dignity of human beings, or the dignity of the human person.

The Hebrew word that is translated as dignity is *gedula.* According to a computer-aided word search, that word occurs only sixteen times in the Hebrew scriptures. It refers to nothing that resembles our contemporary notion of dignity. In general, it refers to rank or position. It doesn't even really refer to nobility of personal character.

The word *dignity* occurs even less frequently in the New Testament. *Aksioprepcia* is not used. The Greek word that is translated as dignity, *semnotes*, may be better translated as "seriousness." There are only three instances that come up on a computer word search—hardly enough to make one take notice. Christian men are urged to "lead a quiet and tranquil life, in dignity" (1 Tim 2:2) and to lead a life characterized by "integrity in your teaching, and dignity" (Tit 2:7). Bishops are admonished to keep their "children under control, with perfect dignity" (1 Tim 3:4).

Thus, it seems fair to say that although scholars may cite the scriptures in support of a particular concept of human dignity, that concept really is a theological theme developed by the church—produced through faithful reflection on revealed truth—rather than something directly revealed through scripture.

Greco-Roman Philosophy

One might suppose, then, that the concept comes down to the twenty-first century through Greek philosophy. Did the Western world inherit the concept of human dignity from the Greeks? The answer is probably not. For Aristotle, at least, dignity (again, in the Greek, *semnotes*) was an acquired virtue, defined as "the mean between servility and unaccomodatingness."[1] Some translators say that *semnotes* may be better rendered as "reserve"—knowing one's place in a social sense. The concept is not even mentioned in the *Nichomachean Ethics*. It also doesn't sound much like what we call dignity today.

Dignity *was* important for the Roman Stoics. One might surmise, then, that if the contemporary notion of dignity did not come from the Greeks, it must have come from the Roman Stoic philosophers. The Latin *dignitas* is most literally translated as "worthiness," which in a political sense meant a man's "reputation or standing." On rare occasions, passages in Cicero refer to the "excellence and dignity of our nature as human beings," but this usage is not typical of Cicero or, in general, of Stoic usage.[2]

Aquinas

Some readers might presume that the theme of human dignity must have originated in the writings of the great Thomas Aquinas. Yet that is not exactly the case either. Granted, making a negative point about Aquinas—considering the sheer volume of his work—is not easy. I have read every one of the nearly 200 instances of the word *dignitas* or its conjugates in the *Summa Theologiae,* however, and Aquinas cannot in any way be construed as the father of the philosophy of human dignity. For Aquinas, dignity was associated with rank. In his hierarchical worldview, everything had a dignity or worth proper to its place. Animals had more dignity than plants, humans had more dignity than animals, men had more dignity than women, kings had more dignity than their subjects, popes had more dignity than kings, and angels had more dignity than popes. This hierarchical view hardly appeals to contemporary audiences, steeped in democratic thought. It seems even less appealing to women. This kind of ranking is not what we seem to mean by dignity today.

Nevertheless, there are two phrases in Aquinas that seem to anticipate the contemporary notion of dignity: *dignitatem hominis* and *dignitas humanae naturae*. These phrases are exceptional, however, and they hardly represent a central concept in his work.[3] In one key passage, Aquinas makes a point in defense of the practice of mystical prayer. He writes, "It belongs to the mode and the dignity of man to be uplifted to the divine because man was created in the image and likeness of God."[4]

This usage has a more familiar ring to contemporary ears, especially to Roman Catholics. On the other hand, one probably could proof-text almost any idea by citing single sentences from the *Summa*. The fact is that this theme of dignity simply is not a major concern for Aquinas.

The Renaissance

The Renaissance brought significant challenges to the view that human beings held an exalted place in the universe. After Copernicus, human dignity simply could no longer depend on human beings' centrality in the cosmos. Perhaps the pivotal figure in the transition to the modern notion of dignity was an Italian, Pico della Mirandola, whose famous oration "On the Dignity of Man" first identified the dignity of human beings with human freedom.[5] As Pico said, "the ability to share in the properties of all other beings, according to his free choice" made human beings exalted.

Pico imagined that God had told human beings, "Fashion thyself in whatever shape thou wilt prefer." This Renaissance view of dignity has had ramifications down to the present.

Hobbes or Kant?

The notion of dignity becomes even more confused by the time of Hobbes. Hobbes had no use for medieval views and even less esteem for Pico. He wrote, "The public worth of a man, which is the value set on him by the Commonwealth, is that which men commonly call DIGNITY."[6]

This view, of course, makes sense if one believes, as Hobbes did, that human life is nothing more than "a perpetual and restless desire of power after power, that ceaseth only in death."[7] Most people, however, do not hold such a view of life (or at least are unwilling to admit that they do). Dignity has a more positive meaning for the modern world.

The Hobbesian view seems to have horrified Kant. In a passage that seems to be a direct response to Hobbes, Kant wrote, "The respect I bear others or which another can claim from me, is the acknowledgement of the dignity of another man, i.e., a worth that has no price, no equivalent for which the object of value could be exchanged. Judging something to have no worth is contempt."[8]

For Kant, not only is human dignity beyond price, it is rooted in the human capacity for free moral choice: "Man's duty to himself insofar as he is a moral being alone . . . consists in the conformity of the maxims of his will with the dignity of the humanity in his person . . . lying, avarice, and false humility contradict the character of man as a moral being, i.e., the internal freedom, the innate dignity of man."[9]

One ought carefully to note, however, the shift in the notion of freedom from the Renaissance to Kant. Pico's type of freedom is largely freedom of choice—freedom as license. Kantian freedom is oriented to moral goodness.

Kant also "democratized" the concept of dignity in a way that Aquinas, given his historical situation, could not. Kant writes, bluntly, "Humanity itself is a dignity."[10]

A Definition of Dignity

Although in the foregoing subsections I offer a broad overview of the history of the word *dignity*, I have not offered a definition. The word appears in countless books and essays today. It has great appeal. In the history I have traced, one learns some idea of where it comes from and about how contemporary usage differs from all sorts of previous historical usages. But what does it mean, exactly?

One can approach a philosophical definition of dignity by evoking the universal experience of human beings as moral agents. Recognition and respect for the intrinsic dignity of human beings can be understood as the fundamental basis of morality. I suggest that a concept akin to that of the dignity of the human person is at the heart of every answer anyone has ever given to the question, why be moral? One can argue that no coherent moral system that recognizes such things as human equality and civil rights, no system that holds a place for war crimes, crimes against humanity, and human rights abuses can hold these positions independent of a recognition of the existence of intrinsic human dignity.

The Rev. Dr. Martin Luther King Jr. recognized this point. He said he learned it from his grandmother, who taught him, simply, "Martin, don't let anyone ever tell you that you're not a somebody."[11] That is the fundamental meaning of intrinsic human dignity: Somebodyness—the conviction that everybody is a somebody.

Pain, Social Worth, Self-Esteem, Control, and Subjective Accounts

If everybody is a somebody, diminutions in pleasure do not make a somebody a nobody. Nor does pleasure make one more of a somebody. Suffering does not make someone a nobody. Being somebody is primary. If one is in pain and wants to be pain-free, one wants to be a pain-free somebody.

Against Hobbes, having no attribution of social worth does not make a somebody into a nobody. Calling someone "a nobody" is a term of derision. In one's heart of hearts, one knows that true morality holds all such assertions false. Everybody is a somebody. Being somebody is more important than what one can contribute to society. If this were not true, there would be no concept of civil rights.

Nor do diminutions in self-esteem make a somebody a nobody. Being somebody is more important than thinking of oneself as important. If this were not true, psychiatrists would not treat people who are suicidally depressed.

Nor can one say that all dignity is subjective. There must be a sense in which everyone knows that everyone else has dignity in advance of an interpersonal encounter and that each has moral responsibilities toward the other even before either party explains what dignity means to him or her. Each human being has an objective place in the manifold goodness of the world. I recognize that I must protect and respect the intrinsic dignity of every person even before any of them tells me anything about what dignity means to him or to her.

The thorniest question for modern Westerners is the relationship between control and dignity. For many, dignity seems to mean being in control. Losing one's valued independence, through the limitations imposed by society or disease—especially by neurological diseases like Lou Gehrig's disease or Alzheimer's disease—seems to mean loss of dignity.

I do not deny that loss of control means loss of the dignity we attribute to other persons. I insist, however, that there is an aspect of dignity that I have called *intrinsic* dignity that remains even when one has lost independence and control.[12] This intrinsic dignity, this being a somebody, is more important than being in control.

Being in control cannot be the definition of dignity. It should be obvious that some of the most important things that happen to anyone—such as one's coming to be at all, or one's inevitable death, or being loved—are entirely out of one's control. The drive to be in control is unrealistic. The deepest aspects of human dignity have nothing to do with control.

This understanding is reflected in common morality. My favorite artistic depiction of intrinsic human dignity is the famous photo of Martin Luther King Jr. in his Birmingham, Alabama, prison cell. He had been denied freedom. He had been denied control. He had been denied dignity by attribution. At times, he must have doubted his own dignity. Yet his intrinsic dignity persisted, simply because he was human. His dignity cried out for recognition. His humanity cried out for justice. Freedom and control are not all there is to dignity.

The crux of the matter is this: We respect the freedom of persons because they have intrinsic dignity. People do not have intrinsic dignity to the extent that they are free. Dignity is more fundamental than freedom. That is why one is not free to dispose of it or to decide for oneself what it means.

Thus, one ought to reject all competing conceptions of human dignity that are based on pleasure, subjectivity, social worth, or freedom and control. By a process of elimination, one arrives at the following alternative.

Intrinsic human dignity means that human beings have a worth and value beyond price, simply because they are human. To say that human dignity consists of something else—of some characteristic that some of us have and some of us do not, or that some of us have more of than others—leads to unacceptable conclusions. Furthermore, if human beings have dignity simply because they are human, the following statements also are true:

- Everyone, by definition, has dignity. Dignity is supremely *democratic*.
- Dignity is truly *inalienable*. No person and no circumstance can take dignity away from any human being.
- Dignity also is truly *qualitative*. It does not admit of degrees. It is the same for everyone.

Attributed versus Intrinsic Dignity

Some readers will rightly object that a homeless schizophrenic who has become demented and is dying alone in the streets has lost his dignity. I do acknowledge that, in a sense, this observation is undeniably true. The confusion can be explained, however, if one takes note of a distinction I draw between *attributed* dignity and *intrinsic* dignity. The kind of dignity I discuss above is *intrinsic* dignity. It is the kind of dignity people have simply because they are members of the human family. It is the dignity that is *intrinsic* to being human.

This kind of dignity may be contrasted with attributed dignity. Attributed dignity is the value or worth one attributes to others or to oneself. It is based on one's power, one's prestige, one's function, one's productivity, and one's degree of control over one's situation. We attribute this sort of dignity to heads of state, for instance, calling them "dignitaries." This sort of dignity is situational—it depends on one's station in life. It differs from person to person, society to society. It changes over time. It can be completely subjective (i.e., how much dignity we are willing to attribute to ourselves) or intersubjective (e.g., how much dignity a society is willing to attribute to its sanitation workers).

Illness and death undeniably attack our *attributed* dignity. Sick people are robbed of their station in life. They become less productive or even unproductive. They lose control. They become dependent. They lose esteem in the eyes of others. Sickness brings this upon them. The central question about dignity and health care, however, is whether such an assault is ultimate and complete or whether there is, after all, such a thing as intrinsic human dignity that can be found even in sickness and death.

There certainly is a moral duty to uphold the attributed dignity of human beings wherever possible. The point is that loss of attributed dignity does not rob a person of intrinsic human dignity. The impetus to reach out and heal is predicated on the notion that persons whom illness has robbed of their station in life are worthy of our concern. That worthiness is their intrinsic dignity. This is how personhood and dignity are related: To be a person is to have intrinsic dignity.

Vulnerability

What of vulnerability? What does that word mean, and what is its relationship to dignity? I suggest that the relationship between these two concepts is profound. In a moral sense, to be vulnerable, simply put, means that the affirmation of one's intrinsic dignity is at risk. Thus, vulnerability is the soft underbelly of personhood. To be vulnerable means that there is a substantial risk that one's worth or value, one's standing as an equal member of the human community, will not be recognized and affirmed.

One obviously is vulnerable when one's life is at stake—when one's very existence as a human being is at risk. One also is vulnerable, however, when one's personhood is at risk in *any* sense—when there is a danger that one will be regarded as no longer equal, no longer counted, no longer worthy of concern.

Thus, the persons who are most vulnerable, particularly in a health care system, are those whose dignity already has been called into question by society before they ever enter the office, clinic, or emergency room—homeless persons, those living with HIV, injection drug users, retarded persons, demented persons, undocumented aliens, and others. Anyone whose worth has been ascribed to anything other than being a member of the human community is vulnerable. Those whose attributed dignity has been assaulted are most at risk for believing that their own intrinsic dignity has been vanquished. This risk applies, above all, to persons who are sick and dying.

Responding to Vulnerability

How ought one respond to the vulnerability of others? Does morality require anything of human beings with respect to their mutual vulnerability?

I believe that the only proper response to vulnerability is love. Love is a dangerous word in philosophy or theology. Yet a Christian cannot escape using it in describing the spiritual life. In love, one puts one's own person at risk—exposing one's own dignity for possible rejection, disappointment, and even possibly annihilation. Love requires exposure of the soft underbelly of one's person. The vulnerability of another requires a response in love—and love requires vulnerability.

Vulnerability is at the core of love because love requires risks. Love means, at the least, exposing oneself to the risk of rejection. It means focusing on the needs of another and thereby forgoing some of one's own (often unconscious and reflexive) self-protective mechanisms. If another human being has been made vulnerable and one reaches out in genuine love, one is thereby also made vulnerable.

I can best illustrate this point with a story. Early in my internship year, I cared for a patient with advanced breast cancer who had developed a pleural effusion (fluid between her lungs and her chest wall) as a result of the spread of her cancer. She certainly was dying, but she was awake and alert and having great difficulty breathing because of the effusion. We decided that she needed to have the fluid removed by a procedure called thoracentesis. In thoracentesis, the skin is anesthetized and a needle is inserted through the chest wall, between the ribs. A small plastic catheter is inserted through the needle and attached to a syringe, and the fluid is drained. When the appropriate amount of fluid has been drained, the catheter is removed. In my patient's case, this procedure had a palliative purpose: Removing the fluid would help her shortness of breath. The oncology fellow asked me to perform the procedure.

As a medical student I had seen this procedure done a few times, and I had helped to perform it once, but I had never done one on my own. Clearly, however, the fellow expected as a matter of course that I was already quite skilled in this procedure. Fearful of seeming less skilled than expected, I answered, "Sure," and proceeded to prepare the equipment to perform the procedure.

I spoke to my patient, explained what we planned to do and why, obtained her written consent, and proceeded to perform the thoracentesis. With a slight give, the needle penetrated into the space where the cancerous fluid was located, and a straw-colored liquid flowed effortlessly back into the syringe. The patient appeared comfortable, with no pain or additional shortness of breath.

I breathed a sigh of relief. I had done it.

I next proceeded to thread the sterile plastic catheter through the needle so that I could take off a large volume of fluid. We thought the patient needed to have at least one, or maybe even two, liters of fluid removed to make her feel more comfortable. As I was inserting the catheter, however, the flow of liquid suddenly stopped. Thinking that the catheter might have become kinked, I pulled it back into the needle to try to reposition it. The catheter seemed to be stuck for a second, then suddenly came back easily. A moment later, the catheter was out of the needle and I realized that the end of it had sheared off somewhere into the fluid filled space between her lungs and her chest.

I broke into a sweat. "How are you doing there?" I asked.

"Just fine," she replied. "It doesn't even hurt a bit. You're a great doctor."

I wasn't sure how to respond. I blurted out, "Well, for some reason the flow of the fluid has stopped. I'm afraid we didn't get much out, and this may not have helped so much. But we're going to have to stop."

"O.K.," she said. "You're the doctor."

My heart was pounding in my chest. What had I done? I should never have tried this without more supervision. Not only was I stupid, I was clumsy. I had visions of the plastic floating around in there. I wondered if its jagged edge might get stuck somewhere between her chest wall and lung and cause a puncture. Maybe it would become infected. I wondered what I could do or should do.

I ordered an X-ray (which was standard after such a procedure anyway), and with trembling hand I paged the fellow.

I remember vividly how kind the fellow was. I had expected an upbraiding, but he was calm and constructive. He told me first things first: The patient was stable and at least for now seemed no worse for the wear. We looked at the X-ray together, and the catheter tip was just sitting there at the bottom of her lung cavity. He told me that everybody makes mistakes and that I should not be too hard on myself. He told me I should make this a learning opportunity—first, that I should never be afraid to ask questions or ask for help out of fear of what someone else might think of me, especially when my reticence put patients at risk. Second, in this specific case, one should never pull back on this type of catheter, whether it is inserted into a body cavity or a vein, because the design makes shearing off the tip very likely.

The fellow said that he wasn't sure himself what to do about it and thought that we should consult a lung specialist who might be able to insert a lighted scope and remove it. After that, we would have to talk to the patient about what had happened.

Talk to the patient? I thought to myself. Is he kidding? All I need is to be sued in the second month of my internship year.

"Can we wait until after the pulmonary consult?" I asked, stalling for time and trying to get my wits about me.

"Sure," he said.

So I waited.

The pulmonologist, Dr. Tsang, was an older Asian man of few words and superb technical skills. Everyone in the hospital regarded him as something of a clinical sage. He looked at the X-rays, looked at the patient, and then said to the fellow and to me, "No problem. Inert material. She die of cancer with plastic sitting there or die of cancer after I take it out. Not worth taking out. No problem. Have nice day."

For a brief moment I was ecstatic. I would not be responsible for her death. It wasn't so serious after all. Then, in the ebb and flow of my emotional riptide, I realized that I still had to talk to the patient. I was terrified once again.

"Do you want me to go with you when you tell her what has happened?" the fellow asked.

"Yes," I said. "I think your presence in the room might help her, and I know it will help me."

"But you'll do the talking, O.K.?"

"Alright," I said. "I'll do the talking."

I was extraordinarily nervous. The overhead fluorescent lights had been switched off, and the room was dimly lit by soft, incandescent bulbs. My palms were cool and sweaty as I sat down beside the patient's bed. The fellow stood behind me, closer to the door. She will think I'm incompetent, I thought. She'll be angry. I'll offer to transfer her case to another intern. She'll sue anyway. My career will be over before it starts. Regardless, I'm just so embarrassed.

"I'm sorry," I started, muttering through trembling lips.

Then I just kept talking. Five minutes of monologue must have passed in which the room seemed to separate itself from time. All that mattered was in this room and was happening at this moment. I must have said "I'm sorry" a dozen times, in a dozen ways. I explained what I had done, what had happened, and why. I told the patient that the pulmonary consultant had recommended just leaving it there.

Then came the patient's turn to speak. I realized that most of my words until this moment had been a way of avoiding what I feared most—her response.

Yet my patient must have been trained by the same mystic guru that had trained Dr. Tsang.

"I'm dying anyway," she said, "so I guess it really doesn't matter, does it, doctor? I'm sure these things happen. Thank you for telling me. But there's really no need for all these apologies. I know you were trying to help me. I know you did your best."

I touched her hand, and we both began to cry. She wiped her tears with a tissue and then, with a small, embarrassed laugh, she offered one to me.

"Thank you," I said, smiling and flushed, with the taste of salt on my lips.

The fellow and I quietly left the room.

A week later she was dead, gone to heaven with a piece of plastic inside her chest—a keepsake from her intern.

I tell this story to illustrate the vulnerability that love for patients requires. I learned this lesson early enough in my career, at least in part through this experience, and I am grateful for it. Trying to escape my vulnerability had gotten me into trouble, and only through embracing that vulnerability could I get myself out of trouble. Real respect for my patient demanded honesty and vulnerability.

Love for patients is always an exercise in vulnerability. The idea is radical and dangerous. Yet it is essential to genuine spirituality in health care.

The Vulnerability of the Healer

To reach out to *any* sick person is to reach out to one who is vulnerable, precisely because his or her dignity is at risk. Is this reaching out an act of love? Is it truly mutual vulnerability?

Although it may not seem obvious, the answer is yes. Healers put their own dignity at risk. They put their own meaning and value and their standing as persons at risk. They are vulnerable in many ways.

First, there often is physical risk. For example, there is the risk of contracting an infectious disease, whether the common cold or the Ebola virus. This is not the stuff of novels only but of genuine reality. I even recall a fellow intern whose Achilles tendon was severed by a "crash cart" while she was running to a "code."

Second, there is interpersonal risk. For example, there is the risk of rejection by the patient or family. Even if one is not "fired," one risks ingratitude on the part of the patient and even, at times, hostility. This rejection is very difficult.

Third, there is the risk of failure. One has offered oneself as a helper. One has presented oneself as certifiably competent. Even the best fail, however, or make mistakes. Ultimately, no one is immortal, and every healer must humbly admit the limits of his or her craft. This vulnerability is profound.

Fourth, there is medico-legal risk. This risk seems to be the only one some health care professionals understand. Every health care professional is vulnerable. One has offered oneself as trustworthy. One might be negligent. One might even be unjustly accused.

Finally (the crux of what makes caring for persons who are *socially* vulnerable so difficult), the most basic vulnerability in healing is the fact that treating another person with respect for that person's intrinsic dignity is to make that person one's equal in the most radical way possible. When any health care professional—nurse, emergency medical technician, psychologist, chaplain, or physician—understands this equality, he or she understands what it means to be vulnerable. Everything about the contemporary health care professional—the degrees, the white coats, the houses, the cars, the published papers, the esteem of the community—is cast aside. When one removes the smelly socks of a homeless person, one makes oneself vulnerable. What such an action communicates is that this person is worthy of one's service, and all the trappings that seem to separate the patient from the health care professional are of lesser value. One can be no more vulnerable than this: recognizing the radical equality of the intrinsic worth of such a person and oneself. There is no other reason to reach out and offer to help—no other reason to try to mitigate the assaults on a patient's attributed dignity, whether wrought by society, fate, the other person's own prior choices, or disease—than the recognition that the patient has dignity that makes him or her worthy of one's service. If the patient's value can be called into question, so can one's own.

This vulnerability is not an overidentification with the suffering of the patient that is so intense that it renders one as helpless as the patient. Neither is it a cold and unfeeling distance, however, or an objectification of the patient as a way of coping with his or her predicament. The patient deserves more than an automaton dispensing technology. The patient also deserves more than a weepy mess for a doctor or nurse. The burned-out health care professional helps no one. I am recommending that the health care professional recognize the unique vulnerability of the patient, ever mindful of the special vulnerability that comes from being one who truly gives *care*.

Vulnerable Persons in Health Care

I now return to the challenge raised by the nurse in the church basement in New Jersey whom I quote at the beginning of this chapter. Why *should* anyone pick a homeless schizophrenic up off the streets of Newark? One does so for the same reason that one picks a Wall Street executive up off the floor of the private bathroom in his office suite: because he or she has intrinsic human dignity. He or she has worth or value, despite whatever situation or situations have placed that dignity at risk. That is to say, each has dignity despite having become vulnerable. Why does one mitigate the assaults on the attributed dignity of each? Because one recognizes each as a fellow human being, bearing the stamp of intrinsic dignity. Persons whose station in life has called their intrinsic dignity into question are at great risk that health care professionals will not respond to their needs. When society has called the intrinsic dignity of a class of persons into question, they enter the health care system already vulnerable, and health care professionals will be preconditioned to regard them as unworthy of their service.

The Social Gospel in New Jersey

I am proud of my Franciscan brothers in New Jersey. I went home to Washington after defending their plans to modify the use of their friary. They persisted in their plans despite the wrath of the local community and fought to open the AIDS hospice. They received threatening phone calls. Their car tires were slashed. They attended public hearings and fought against legal maneuvers designed to thwart them in the courts. They took these risks. They became vulnerable. I believe they did it for love.

The AIDS hospice finally opened. Although advances in HIV treatment have led to changes in this old friary's mission, people living with HIV are still being served there today.

Difficult Patients

Vulnerability in health care comes in many forms. Health care professionals sometimes do not like to admit it, but there are always patients for whom they do not like to provide care. Psychoanalysts may attribute much of this reluctance to countertransference—the way these patients might remind their doctors or nurses of a wicked stepmother or some other painful but significant relationship. Although this factor may be at least a partial explanation in many cases, much of this phenomenon is linked to the notion of vulnerability and how health professionals deal with it. So-called difficult patients typically are either hostile, or ungrateful, "noncompliant," or "self-abusive."

Caring for these patients is very difficult because the healer receives so little in return for the services rendered. If the patient does not seem to take his or her own dignity seriously, why should the health care professional bother? The whole process can seem futile. Often, nothing changes. The forces that have placed the patient in such a horrific situation can seem insurmountable. The doctor or nurse may feel like the little Dutch Boy with his finger in the dike holding back the sea of insoluble social problems. The physician may feel like Sisyphus, writing pre-

scriptions that the patient will not take. The nurse may feel the pangs
of unrequited love when her attentive care is greeted with insults in
return.

Certainly there are many things one can do to try to address these
issues. There are ways to improve compliance. Social workers can help
arrange services for patients to mitigate difficult social situations. If the
patient has features of a borderline personality disorder, one can prevent "splitting" by unifying the staff response and setting clear limits on
patient behavior. If one is vulnerable enough to be humble, however,
ultimately one must admit that there are many things that health care
simply cannot do. Social science cannot eliminate all noncompliance.
Not all patients will love their doctors and nurses, thank them, and
bake them cookies for Christmas. Neither individually nor collectively
will health care professionals ever eradicate the poverty, ignorance, and
social injustice that breed so much of the disease they treat. Patients
will always mistrust them and insult them.

Caring for difficult patients is not easy. It may help to remind health
care professionals that such patients have intrinsic dignity as well. Dignity is the worth that has no price, that all patients have—whether dirty
or clean, rich or poor, expected to recover or expected to die, grateful
or ungrateful, compliant or noncompliant.

One puts one's own dignity on the line when one cares for anyone,
but especially in caring for these patients. Yet their dignity is our dignity—a worth beyond price. Their vulnerability is our vulnerability—
the context and the signature of healing. Veterinarians may be able to
cure cats and horses. Only persons, however, can heal persons.[13]

Notes

1. Aristotle, *Eudemian Ethics*, 2nd ed.,1221a.8, trans. Michael Woods (New
York: Oxford University Press, 1991), 17.

2. Cicero, *De Officiis*, trans. Walter Miller (Cambridge, Mass.: Loeb Classical
Library, Harvard University Press, 1975), 108–9.

3. Thomas Aquinas, *Summa Theologiae*, Blackfriars ed., II-II, q. 84, a.1, ad.1;
III, q.1, ad. 2 (New York: McGraw-Hill, 1963).

4. Ibid., II-II, q. 175, a.1, ad.2.

5. Giovanni Piccolo della Mirandola, *De Hominis Dignitate,* Italian translation and commentary by Giovanni Semprini (Rome: Editrice Atranor, 1986).

6. Thomas Hobbes, *Leviathan,* X, ed. Richard Tuck (Cambridge: Cambridge University Press, 1991), 63–64.

7. Ibid., XI, 70.

8. Immanuel Kant, "The Metaphysics of Morals, part II: The Metaphysical Principles of Virtue," Ak419–20, in *Ethical Philosophy,* trans. James W. Ellington (Indianapolis: Hackett, 1983), 80–81.

9. Ibid., Ak462, 127.

10. Ibid.

11. Garth Baker-Fletcher, *Somebodyness: Martin Luther King, Jr. and the Theory of Dignity,* Harvard Dissertations in Divinity, no. 31 (Minneapolis: Fortress Press, 1993), 23.

12. Daniel P. Sulmasy, "Death and Human Dignity," *Linacre Quarterly* 61, no. 4 (1994): 27–36; Daniel P. Sulmasy, "Death with Dignity: What Does It Mean?" *Josephinum Journal of Theology* 4 (1997): 13–24.

13. Abraham Joshua Heschel, *The Insecurity of Freedom* (New York: Noonday Press/Farrar, Strauss, Giroux, 1966), 24–38.

The Wisdom of Ben Sira

I n the first three chapters of this book I discuss the experiential basis for calling health care a spiritual practice. I now turn to an ancient text to look for spiritual wisdom. As I argue in chapter 2, even nonbelievers ought to accept that religious traditions are wisdom traditions and that they contain spiritual insights that can be helpful to all practitioners and patients. The text I examine in this chapter is far older than the modern scientific clinic. It contains ancient wisdom that might help health care professionals today rediscover how scientific medicine and spirituality can be integrated once again.

Discomfort regarding the relationship between spirituality and scientific medicine is not a new phenomenon. Ancient peoples sensed this tension, even if they came at the question from a position of skepticism about science rather than skepticism about spirituality. Ancient religious texts can help illuminate our struggles, provide advice, and suggest solutions that will be relevant even in the twenty-first century. Through analysis of one such ancient text, "The Wisdom of Ben Sira," I explore in more detail how the spiritual aspirations of patients and clinicians can be drawn together in a covenantal understanding of health care.

This ancient text is sometimes referred to as "The Physician's Prayer," yet it has not received much scholarly attention and rarely has been presented to health care professionals in a format that would enable them to understand its historical and religious significance and

44

possible relevance to their own work today. The text arises out of Jewish spirituality, in contact with ancient Greek medicine. I believe it contains important messages for contemporary health care.

The Text

"The Wisdom of Ben Sira," also variously known as "The Proverbs of Ben Sira," "*Liber Ecciesiasticus*," "*Ecclesiasticus*," and "Sirach," probably was composed around 180 BCE.[1] The text originally was composed in Hebrew (as corroborated by textual evidence from Qumran and other archeological sites) and later was translated into Greek, Syriac, and eventually Latin.[2]

Although this text was recognized from the earliest Christian times as divinely inspired, modern Protestants and Jews consider the book Deuterocanonical, or part of the Apocrypha. It seems certain that it was included in a loose collection of writings considered sacred by first-century Palestinian Jews. About 100 CE, however, after the destruction of Jerusalem, the rabbinical community decided to designate a portion of those sacred writings as part of an official canon. This text—which by then had been accepted as divinely inspired by the already distinct Christian community—was excluded from the official Jewish canon. Nevertheless, Ben Sira is quoted eighty-two times in the Talmud and related Jewish writings of the first few centuries CE.[3] Even today, Jewish writing about medical ethics cites Ben Sira.[4] Although the Roman Catholic Church still upholds the canonicity of Ben Sira's book, the leaders of the Protestant Reformation preached a return to the Jewish canon and excluded Ben Sira's writings from their Bible.[5]

"The Wisdom of Ben Sira" is counted among the other books of the "wisdom" literature in the scriptures, such as Proverbs, Job, The Wisdom of Solomon, and Qoholeth or Ecclesiastes.[6] The following translation of the first fifteen verses of the thirty-eighth chapter from the New Revised Standard Version (NRSV) Bible is the text I explore in this chapter:

1. Honor physicians for their services, for the Lord created them;
2. for their gift of healing comes from the Most High, and they are rewarded by the King.
3. The skill of physicians makes them distinguished, and in the presence of the great they are admired.
4. The Lord created medicines out of the earth, and the sensible will not despise them.
5. Was not water made sweet with a tree in order that His power might be known?
6. And He gave skill to human beings that He might be glorified in His marvelous works.
7. By them the physician heals and takes away pain;
8. the pharmacist makes a mixture from them. God's works will never be finished; and from Him health spreads over all the earth.
9. My child, when you are ill, do not delay, but pray to the Lord, and He will heal you.
10. Give up your faults and direct your hands rightly, and cleanse your heart from all sin.
11. Offer a sweet-smelling sacrifice, and a memorial portion of your choice flour, and pour oil on your offering as much as you can afford.
12. Then give the physician his place, for the Lord created him; do not let him leave you, for you need him.
13. There may come a time when recovery lies in the hands of physicians,
14. for they too pray to the Lord, that He grant them success in diagnosis, and in healing, for the sake of preserving life.
15. He who sins against his Maker will be defiant toward the physician.

The Author

The author's full name was Joshua (or Jesus) ben Eleazar ben Sira.[7] He was trained as a scribe, traveled extensively, and settled in Jerusalem, where he probably taught in some sort of school for young men. His grandson later migrated to Egypt and translated "The Wisdom of Ben Sira" into Greek. Little else can be said about the author's life.[8]

Sociocultural Influences

The history of the Near East has always been stormy. The three centuries preceding the birth of Christ were no exception to this rule. Alexander the Great defeated the Persians in 332 BCE. The conquerors brought their culture with them into Palestine, and a period of profound Greek influence ensued. After Alexander's death in 322 BCE, two of his generals fought for control of the area. The victor crowned himself Ptolemy I of Egypt. The loser, Seleucus, kept control of what is now Syria. After several generations of rule by Egyptian kings of the Ptolemaic Dynasty, the Seleucids gained control of Palestine in 198 BCE. The ambitious Seleucids tried to extend their empire into Greece, but there they met defeat at the hands of the Romans in 190 BCE. Although the Seleucids maintained control over Palestine for some time after this defeat, they were severely weakened by the burdensome peace terms imposed by the Romans.[9]

This period in Jewish history is known as the period of "Hellenization." Through most of what we suspect to be the lifetime of Ben Sira, as long as they paid their heavy taxes and did not rebel, for the most part the Jews were allowed to keep their own customs and laws.[10] Sometime after the death of Ben Sira the more forceful program of Hellenization enacted by later Seleucid kings gave rise to the Maccabean revolt in 166 BCE.[11]

Nonetheless, the sociocultural impact of Hellenism was profound. The Jews had "a gnawing, unexpressed fear that the religion of their ancestors was inadequate to cope with the needs of social and political structures that were changed enormously."[12] These were the times of Ben Sira. Rationalistic Greek philosophy and science challenged Jewish scholarship and threatened Jewish identity. "In general, Ben Sira is a representative of Palestinian Jewry in the process of redefining its position face to face with an increasing Hellenistic influence."[13] As part of their response to Hellenistic influence, Jewish authors created a category of "inspired learning" in which wise men acquired prophetic features and prophets came to be regarded as wise men.[14] Jewish wisdom literature arose in this period. We must understand the text from Ben

Sira in this context. Like so many other elements in the life of the Palestinian Jew of the second century BCE, Greek wisdom and Jewish tradition were in conflict regarding the meaning of medicine and the role it ought to play in society. What was the nature of this conflict, and how could it be resolved?

Medicine and Medical Ethics in Jewish History and in the Wisdom of Ben Sira

Before the time of Ben Sira there was no medical profession per se among the Jews.[15] Jews apparently did not even have their own embalmers; according to Genesis 50:2–3, they had to ask the Egyptians to embalm Jacob.[16] The Hebrew word for physician is *rophi*. For Jews, God was Rophi Cholim, "the Supreme Physician."[17] "I, the Lord, am your Healer" (Ex. 15:25). In Deuteronomy 32:39 one reads, "It is I who bring both death and life, I who inflict wounds and heal them, and from my hand there is no rescue." Illness could be created only by God as a direct act, and only God could heal.[18] The term *rophi* usually was used pejoratively in the Hebrew Scriptures. Physicians were magicians and idol-worshipers, and pious Jews could have nothing to do with them.[19] God alone could heal. King Asa was chastised for appealing to physicians for a cure instead of turning to God (2 Chron. 16:12–13).

Certainly Jews practiced at least some medicine. Hampered by the lack of texts on the subject of medicine from this period, contemporary understanding of just what second-century BCE Jewish medicine was like is very limited.[20] The Hebrew Scriptures make reference to a small number of pharmaceuticals, such as mandrake root for infertility (Gen. 30:14), a metaphorical salve for Israel's wounds (Is. 1:6), a scarcity of balm in Gilead (Jer. 8:22), an inefficacious plaster of figs for the King's boil (2 Kings 20:7–27), and fish gall for the eyes of the blind (Tob. 11:12). There also is evidence from the scrolls uncovered at Qumran that the Essenes—very roughly contemporaries of Ben Sira—practiced a significant amount of medicine. In fact, their name can be rendered as "Healers."[21] Some of these scrolls contain stories of angels revealing secret herbal cures to Noah. The Essenes seem to have had no direct influence, however, from the Greek medicine being practiced at the time in Alexandria.[22] The Qumran community had two types of practitioners, *therapeutae* and *hemerobaptists*. Both types included prayer in all of their cures.[23] The bulk of evidence, however, suggests that Jewish medicine was underdeveloped before the time of Ben Sira. "Israelite medical expertise was virtually restricted to the treatment of external injuries. . . . It is [therefore] reasonable to suppose that the growing interest in medical science" which is noted in the time of Ben Sira must be ascribed to innovations of foreign origin.[24]

What were some of these foreign innovations? From the most ancient times, prior to the Greek conquest, Jews were strongly influenced by the empires to their east. The fish gall used in the Book of Tobit is mentioned elsewhere in Assyrian writings.[25] From Babylon came a mixture of empiricism and a medical practice based on the presumption that all disease was caused by demonic possession and required incantations as well as herbal pharmaceuticals for treatment.[26] "Like the Babylonians, the Jews attributed healing and sickness to God. Unlike them, priests were not healers. The Jewish priests performed temple rituals and inspections of the sick, but did not perform cures."[27] Moreover, despite much modern effort to ascribe hypothetical public health benefits to practices such as Jewish dietary laws and rituals of the "clean" and the "unclean," one must remember that the overwhelming and primary purpose of these laws was spiritual. Any public health benefit that accrued was largely incidental.[28]

Egyptian influence on Jewish medicine also was significant, even from very ancient times. The concept of a "pneumatic" life principle (Gen. 7:22 and 1 Kings 17:17–22) seems to have had Egyptian origins.[29] Circumcision—originally a ritual reserved for the priestly class of Egyptians—became the only known surgery performed by ancient Jews, thus consecrating them as a "priestly people."[30] In the Hellenistic period, much of the "new wisdom" in Israel came via Egypt. Ancient Egyptian papyri describing a 500-item apothecary are known to have existed at the time of Ben Sira.[31] Egypt at the time of Ben Sira overflowed with physicians.[32] Prominent among them was a neo-Pythagorean named Bolus (Democritus) of Mendes, who lived from about 250 to 150 BCE. He practiced a Greek style of medicine known as "sympatheia."[33]

Clearly "the great evolution in medical science and the shift of the Greek schools from magic and dogmatic medicine to clinical medicine and the revolutionary changes in medical doctrine and practice . . . were not brought about by Jewish scholars."[34] Yet Jews often were educated through the Greeks at Alexandria during the time of the Ptolemies, especially in medicine.[35]

Greek medicine was not assimilated wholesale into Jewish thought. The humoral theory of the Greeks met with significant skepticism by Jews.[36] One hypothesis is that the Jewish tradition of examining slaughtered animals for evidence of illnesses that would render these animals "unclean" gave rise to a significant understanding of pathological anatomy despite prohibitions on the dissection of human cadavers. Thus, Jewish pathophysiology put a stronger emphasis on organ-localized and "solid" diseases than the corresponding Greek pathophysiology.[37]

Even more important, Jews had to contend with their traditional view that physicians were a degraded lot of magicians and idol-worshippers. How could a pious Jew accept these new Greek ideas about medicine? In some ways, empirical and scientific Greek medicine, divorced from any association with the gods or religion, provided the first opportunity for Jews to understand medicine freed from the ritual contamination of magic and worship of false gods. For example, the Hippocratic *De Morbo Sacro*, a treatise on epilepsy, specifically condemns magical views regarding this disease in a way with which a Jew could certainly identify.[38] The ethics of the Hippocratic oath also were congenial to Jewish thought.[39] For the first time, Jews could read medical treatises that condemned magical views of medicine as strongly as any rabbi. Now, however, something new was being offered to take its place: scientific and empirical medicine, which might not be intrinsically sinful.

Even if Jews began to realize that they could practice medicine without participating in magic or worship of alien gods, however, they had a more basic theological problem to deal with. How could a Jew be presumptuous enough to assimilate to himself the power to heal that was, as the scriptures indicate, a power Yahweh reserved to Himself alone? A pious Jew would hesitate to practice medicine or be treated by a doctor.

Acceptance of Religious Legitimacy

Just a few centuries after the writings of Ben Sira, Jewish writings generally reflect acceptance of the religious legitimacy of the medical profession. The Midrash contains stories likening the work of a physician to that of a farmer—not interfering in God's nature, but making use of the gifts given to him by God.[40] The Talmud makes provisions for the use of medical testimony in official Jewish courts and requires both medical licensing and the presence of a physician during the administration of corporal punishment.[41] By the sixth century CE, the oath for Jewish physicians written by Asaph makes clear that physicians had become members of a noble profession that had religious importance but was completely scientific and dissociated from all magic. "He causes healing plants to grow and puts skill to heal into the hearts of sages by his manifold mercies to declare His wonders to the multitudes and to understand all living things, for He was their creator and that apart from Him there is no Savior."[42] The similarities to the thirty-eighth chapter of the Wisdom of Ben Sira are striking enough to make one believe that the Oath of Asaph was influenced by the earlier text.

The justification of the physician's right to heal apparently still was contested in some circles of Jewish thought through the tenth century CE.[43] By the time of Maimonides, however, the Torah's prescription to restore lost objects to one's neighbor (Deut. 22:2) and not to stand idly by the blood of one's fellow (Lev. 19:18) was interpreted as prescribing an actual duty on the part of the physician to heal.[44]

None of these later developments would have been possible, however, without somehow reserving a place for God in the process of diagnosis and healing. A Jew might accept scientific medical practice as not intrinsically disordered, but a detached scientific physician operating apart from God still would have been an abomination. Ben Sira's poem is the earliest known Jewish text to grapple with this problem. Ben Sira offers Jews a reconciliation between Greek medicine and their own tradition. He "insists that the summoning of the medical man . . . in no way indicates a lack of faith in God's ability to heal."[45] When Ben Sira writes (v. 12) "for you need him," he seems to be implying that prayer is not enough. God will still do the healing, but God has ordained things so that God will accomplish healing through the community of human beings. The sick person must turn, at God's insistence, to his "fellow." God will heal, but only in and through and with the doctor, whose profession God has established (v. 1) for this purpose. God, Ben Sira seems to think, will not allow the sick person to be isolated. The patient needs healing from God, but this healing is to be accomplished through the community—first by approaching the temple with sin-offerings (v. 11) and then by seeking out the doctor (v. 12). Thus, in this passage, Ben Sira establishes the right of the physician to heal, not through magic but through knowledge of the sort that the Hellenizers had recently introduced into his homeland: knowledge that had its basis in God. This new understanding was crucial in the history of medicine and Jewish theology. One cannot say whether it originated with Ben Sira or he simply recorded the common wisdom of his day. Certainly, however, the metaphor of the farmer from the Midrash and the Oath of Asaph are similar enough in content to the thirty-eighth chapter of "The Wisdom of Ben Sira" to suspect that this text had a significant impact on later Jewish thought regarding the roles of God and the physician in the work of healing.

Ben Sira also grapples with the notion of "Deuteronomic retribution" that is so deeply embedded in the consciousness of the people of Israel—a theme that recurs repeatedly in the Hebrew Scriptures.[46] Illness usually was considered a result of sin—either one's own sin or that of one's ancestors. Disease or misfortune also could be a sort of test of fidelity to God's covenant. All human fortune—perceived as trial, reward, or punishment—was meted out by God in this life, however, not in any afterlife. Ben Sira accepts this doctrine and does not attempt the kind of sophisticated theodicy found, for example, in Job. Thus, in verses 9–11 Ben Sira insists on the classic triad of prayer, repentance, and sacrifice as the basic prescription for anyone who is sick. In addition, of course, he insists on the importance of the Hellenistic physician and his medicines, but he will not forget his religious roots while prescribing teas concocted from the roots of vegetables.

A Significant Verse

Verse 5 is very significant. It refers to Exodus 15:22–26, where the people of Israel, having left Egypt for the desert, have only bitter water to drink. Moses prays to God, and God responds by showing Moses a tree twig. Moses then casts this tree branch into the waters that suddenly are made drinkable. Ben Sira breaks with the traditional understanding of this event as a *Deus ex machina* miracle.[47] He interprets this twig as a pharmaceutical agent, which already had the power to "cure" the waters inhering in its substance. God created this twig (and presumably many others) to possess such powers. He gives human beings the capability of discovering and unleashing this power. The power and the glory still belong to God, but human beings participate in that power. Note also that this passage from Exodus concludes with one of the aforementioned "problem" texts: "I, the Lord, am your healer."

In an important way, Ben Sira has not only "demythologized" the story of the twig to theologically justify pharmaceutical medicine, he also has given the pious Jew further opportunities to reconcile tradition and the "new medicine." Yahweh still heals—but in and through physicians whom he has endowed with the capability of discovering the healing power that God has already created in the natural world. Ben Sira has cast Moses in the role of the physician. God "cured" the water through Moses. God is still *Rophi Cholim*, but God cures patients through human physicians. Moreover, the physician is not simply a passive instrument through whom God's healing power is channeled. The physician is not static. Strikingly, in verse 8 Ben Sira contends that the physician and the druggist are instruments by whom God actually extends the work of creation. The implication is that through them,

"God's works will never be finished." The physician does not merely
"discover" healing power already in creation but through human imagi-
nation, grounded in divine creativity, makes new healing substances
and new acts of healing. The works of healing and discovering new
medicines (i.e., both "clinical" medicine and "'research" medicine) extend the work of creation—not passively, but dynamically; not miracu-
lously, but humanly.

No wonder, then, that the physician is elevated to such a lofty status
in this text and in so many later Jewish writings on this subject. To
justify the physician's right to heal—a right that traditionally had been
reserved to Yahweh himself—Ben Sira and his successors gave the physician a status nearly at God's right hand. "Honor" is a word used rarely
in "The Wisdom of Ben Sira."[48] It is used to refer to God, to fathers,
to nobility, to ancestors, and to physicians. One also must remember,
however, that at that time every royal court in the Hellenized world
outside of Israel had a court physician.[49] During those times, when
"wisdom had gained possession of every people and nation," physicians
also were beginning to be noted for their particular wisdom.[50] Thus, as
Ben Sira notes in verses 1–3, "honor" is due the physician not only because of a new theologized understanding of the physician but also by
virtue of the physician's status as a member of royal courts, as well as
popular recognition of the extent of the physician's knowledge.

Has Ben Sira simply placed the physician on a pedestal and en-
throned him as a god of healing? Does the lofty status he has assigned
to the physician not border on idol worship? Certainly not. The physician heals only by God's plan and by God's will. The physician must
always recognize this connection to be successful; therefore (v. 13–14),
he also must pray, so that his skills in diagnosis and therapeutics might
truly be "efficacious." There is a sense in which the "therapeutic moment"—the moment in which God's creative power is actualized in the
work of the physician—is a sacred moment for the prayerful practitioner. Adinolfi points out that the Hebrew word 'et ("time") corresponds to the Greek kairos precisely, including the fact that both words
can be understood in two senses: There is a "weak" sense of "generic"
time and a "strong" sense of "right time" or "favorable circumstances."[51]

When Ben Sira writes that "there are times that give him an advantage," one may understand *'et* in this strong sense and realize that the strength of the "right time" is bidirectional. The patient will be healed, and the pious physician himself will experience his share in God's creative power in a unique and prayerful way. The physician himself will be touched by the *Rophi Cholim* and humbled by the experience. The moment can be sacred for both doctor and patient.

What is the patient's role? Must the patient remain a passive recipient of a paternalistic physician's activity? Certainly there is only a limited role for patient "autonomy," as the term is understood by modern authors in the field of biomedical ethics. In the writings of Ben Sira, however, the patient has plenty of responsibility for his or her own health care. This text from the thirty-eighth chapter of "The Wisdom of Ben Sira" follows a long discourse in the thirty-seventh chapter in which the reader is urged to avoid gluttony, which is bound to bring on illness. This sort of admonition is consonant with the writings of Hillel (first century CE), who urged his readers to bathe and care for their bodies because they were created in the image and likeness of God.[52] At many other points Ben Sira urges moderation in all things as the key to health (31:2; 31:22; 37:19; 37:29–30). He begins his book by promising that wisdom makes "peace and perfect health to flourish" (1:18), and he urges a sort of preventive medicine in all aspects of life when he writes, "before you fall ill, take care of your health" (18:19). The patient must not neglect the basic prescription of prayer, repentance, and sacrifice (v. 9–11). The patient must honor the doctor (v. 1), give him his place (v. 12), and not be defiant toward him (v. 15). This requirement, however, is not because the patient is considered an unworthy pawn manipulated by a powerful doctor. Some scholars have translated v. 15 as "Whoever sins against God falls into the hands of the physician."[53] Others, through careful textual study and in an effort to preserve the internal consistency of the entire passage, have translated it as, "He who is a sinner toward his Maker will be defiant toward the physician (doctor)."[54]

If one accepts this latter translation, one can easily see how Ben Sira draws the analogy between Yahweh's relationship with his people and the relationship between doctor and patient. One who is defiant toward God is defiant toward the doctor. Paul Ramsey insists even in our contractual and litigious times, the relationship between doctor and patient is best described by an analogy to the covenant between Yahweh and His people.[55] Ben Sira seems to have had this insight many centuries ago.

William May describes a covenant as a special relationship that entails "duties that give specific content to the future, while enjoining a comprehensive fidelity that extends beyond the particulars to unforeseen and unforeseeable contingencies."[56] This is the kind of relationship Yahweh undertook with the people of Israel: not a *quid pro quo* contract but a covenant. The overall spirit of the relationship between doctor and patient that emerges from Ben Sira's poem also is one of a covenant.

Like the relationship between Yahweh and his people, the relationship between patient and physician may seem tenuous at times. Although Yahweh promised never to abandon the people of Israel, they often wandered far from Yahweh and his law and might even have been led to fear abandonment in retribution for their sins. Likewise a Jewish patient might have feared (v. 12) that the doctor would leave him.

Nonetheless, the picture that emerges is of a covenant nested within a covenant—the physician and patient have a covenant with each other, and their covenantal relationship is grounded in the covenant Yahweh already has with both of them. Both the patient and the physician have responsibilities in relation to one another and to God. The physician's energies and prayers are directed toward the good of the patient—a correct diagnosis and cure (v. 14). The patient prays for healing and forgiveness (v. 9–11) and respects the physician (v. 1, 12). The overarching relationship between God and his people subsumes and sustains the relationship between doctor and patient. The promise of God and the promise of the doctor intersect at the therapeutic moment when repentance meets forgiveness and sickness meets healing. This is the *kairos* of the covenant between doctor and patient. This is the moment in which tradition and Greek science are reconciled. This is the moment of efficacious power and of God's unending creativity. It is the moment Ben Sira saw more than 2,000 years ago—a moment we still struggle to see reborn today.

Notes

1. P. A. Skehan and A. A. DiLella, *The Wisdom of Ben Sira*, Anchor Bible Series, vol. 39 (New York: Doubleday, 1987), 9–10; R. A. F. MacKenzie, *Sirach, Old Testament Message*, vol. 19 (Wilmington, Del.: Michael Glazier, 1983), 13.

2. Skehan and DiLella, *Wisdom of Ben Sira*, 8, 51–62.

3. Ibid., 17–20.

4. E. Bickerman, "The Historical Foundations of Post-Biblical Judaism," in *The Jews: Their History, Culture, and Religion*, 3rd ed., vol. 1, ed. L. Finkelstein (Westport, Conn.: Greenwood Press, 1979), 94; S. Munter, "Medicine in Ancient Israel," in *Medicine in the Bible and Talmud*, ed. F. Rosner (New York: Ktav Publishing, 1977), 3–21.

5. MacKenzie, *Sirach*, 18.

6. Skehan and DiLella, *Wisdom of Ben Sira*, 33.

7. MacKenzie, *Sirach*, 15.

8. Skehan and DiLella, *Wisdom of Ben Sira*, 10–11.

9. Ibid., 12–16.

10. Ibid., 12–14.

11. MacKenzie, *Sirach*, 14.

12. Skehan and Dilella, *Wisdom of Ben Sira*, 16.

13. S. Noorda, "Illness and Sin, Forgiving, and Healing: The Connection of Medical Treatment and Religious Beliefs in Ben Sira 38.15," in *Studies in Hellenistic Religions*, ed. M. J. Vermassen (Leyden, The Netherlands: E. J. Brill, 1979), 215–24.

14. M. Henzel, *Judaism and Hellenism*, vol. 1 (Philadelphia: Fortress Press, 1974), 206.

15. E. N. Dorff, "The Jewish Tradition," in *Caring and Curing: Health and Medicine in the Western Religious Traditions*, ed. R. L. Numbers and D. W. Amundsen (New York: Macmillan, 1986), 15; A. Castiglioni, "The Contribution of the Jews to Medicine," in *The Jews: Their History, Culture, and Religion*, 3rd ed., vol. 2, ed. L. Finkelstein (Westport, Conn.: Greenwood Press, 1979), 1349–75.

16. Castiglioni, "The Contribution of the Jews to Medicine."

17. O. Bettman, *A Pictorial History of Medicine* (Springfield, Ill.: Charles C. Thomas, 1956), 9–10.

18. D. M. Feldman, *Health and Medicine in the Jewish Tradition* (New York: Crossroad, 1986), 15.

19. Castiglioni, "The Contribution of the Jews to Medicine"; Dorff, "The Jewish Tradition"; Noorda, "Illness and Sin, Forgiving, and Healing."

20. S. Munter, "Medicine," in *Encyclopedia Judaica*, vol. 11, ed. C. Roth (Jerusalem: Keter Publishing, 1971), 1178–211.

21. Ibid.
22. Henzel, *Judaism and Hellenism*, vol. 1, 240–41.
23. Castiglioni, "The Contribution of the Jews to Medicine."
24. Noorda, "Illness and Sin, Forgiving, and Healing."
25. G. von Rad, *Wisdom in Israel* (New York: Abingdon Press, 1972), 134–37.
26. M. Adinolfi, "Il Medico in Sir 38, 1–15," *Antonianum* 62 (1987): 173–82; R. K. Harrison, "Medicine in the Bible," in *Interpreter's Dictionary of the Bible*, vol. 3, ed. G. A. Buttrick (New York: Abingdon Press, 1962), 331–34.
27. Munter, "Medicine."
28. Dorff, "The Jewish Tradition," 11.
29. Castiglioni, "The Contribution of the Jews to Medicine."
30. Ibid.
31. Skehan and DiLella, *Wisdom of Ben Sira*, 438–43.
32. Adinolfi, "Il Medico in Sir 38, 1–15."
33. Henzel, *Judaism and Hellenism*, vol. 2, 162, n. 848.
34. Castiglioni, "The Contribution of the Jews to Medicine."
35. Munter, "Medicine"; Castiglioni, "The Contribution of the Jews to Medicine"; J. G. Snaith, *Ecclesiasticus, or the Wisdom of Jesus, Son of Sirach* (New York: Cambridge University Press, 1974), 183–85.
36. Feldman, *Health and Medicine in the Jewish Tradition*, 36.
37. C. D. Spivak, "Medicine in the Bible and Talmud," in *The Jewish Encyclopedia*, vol. 8, ed. I. Singer (New York: Ktav Publishing, 1964), 409–13; Munter, "Medicine."
38. Noorda, "Illness and Sin, Forgiving, and Healing."
39. L. Edelstein, *Ancient Medicine* (Baltimore: Johns Hopkins University Press, 1967), 62–63.
40. Dorff, "The Jewish Tradition," 16; Feldman, *Health and Medicine in the Jewish Tradition*, 15.
41. Spivak, "Medicine in the Bible and Talmud."
42. S. Munter, "Hebrew Medical Ethics and the Oath of Asaph," *Journal of the American Medical Association* 205 (1968): 96–97.
43. F. Rosner, "The Best of Physicians Is Destined for Gehenna," *New York State Journal of Medicine* 83 (1983): 970–72.
44. F. Rosner, *Medicine in the Mishnah Torah of Maimonides* (New York: Ktav Publishing, 1984), 61–67.
45. MacKenzie, *Sirach*, 143.
46. Skehan and DiLella, *Wisdom of Ben Sira*, 83–87, 438–43.
47. Snaith, *Ecclesiasticus*, 184–85; MacKenzie, *Sirach*, 143.
48. Adinolfi, "Il Medico in Sir 38, 1–15."
49. Ibid.; Snaith, *Ecclesiasticus*, 184–85; Skehan and DiLella, *Wisdom of Ben Sira*, 438–43.
50. Bickerman, "Historical Foundations of Post-Biblical Judaism," 94.
51. Adinolfi, "Il Medico in Sir 38, 1–15."

52. Dorff, "The Jewish Tradition," 19.

53. von Rad, *Wisdom in Israel,* 135; Snaith, *Ecclesiasticus,* 184–85.

54. Skehan and DiLella, *Wisdom of Ben Sira,* 438–43; Adinolfi, "Il Medico in Sir 38, 1–15"; Noorda, "Illness and Sin, Forgiving, and Healing."

55. P. Ramsey, *The Patient as Person* (New Haven, Conn.: Yale University Press, 1970), xi–xviii.

56. W. F. May, *The Physician's Covenant: Images of the Healer in Medical Ethics,* 2nd ed. (Louisville, Ky.: Westminster John Knox Press, 2000), 113.

$\sim\!\!\!\odot$ 5

The Dialectic of Healing

I n the preceding chapters I argue that health care is a spiritual practice. I point to the spiritual nature of the experience of practicing the healing professions and look to ancient wisdom literature. In this chapter I attempt to reach the same conclusion by a different method. I lay out philosophical, theological, and historical arguments that health care is essentially spiritual. The method I use is dialectical and Hegelian in structure. In a Hegelian spirit, I offer a philosophical interpretation of human history—limited, however, to the history of spirituality and medicine. The dialectical technique I use also is Hegelian—thesis, antithesis, synthesis. The argument begins not from the spiritual experiences of practitioners or ancient wisdom literature but from the experience each person has of sickness and suffering. This chapter is very different in style and harder to read than the previous chapters. It adds substantially, however, to the themes of this book. Genuine spirituality should not be anti-intellectual. These two approaches are complementary, and the fact that both converge on the same conclusion suggests, by consilience, that this conclusion is true.

Paradoxes of Health Care

Health care is essentially paradoxical. Yet the paradoxes at the heart of health care rarely are appreciated. The first of these paradoxes is that medical practice is both universal and particular. The need to which medicine ministers—the need for healing—is universal to the human condition. Yet medicine can be understood and practiced only on a case-by-case basis in which particular practitioners care for particular patients. Second, the practice of medicine is both subjective and objective. The need for healing undeniably is determined subjectively. Yet illness also obviously manifests itself objectively, and healing is objectively rendered. Third, the goals of medicine are simultaneously infinite and finite. The need to which medicine ministers, the need for healing, ultimately is an infinite need. Yet medicine can be practiced only by finite practitioners with finite skills and finite resources caring for ultimately finite patients.

Hence, the task of medicine appears impossible—an inherently objective, particular, and finite enterprise addressing an inherently subjective, universal, and infinite need. In this chapter I present a dialectical understanding of the apparent paradoxes of medicine as they are made manifest in the doctor-patient relationship. I argue that a proper understanding of medicine requires a spiritual context, or it will remain an irresolvably paradoxical enterprise. I argue that the subjective, universal, and infinite terms that medical practice demands constitute a spiritual field of experience. Any theory of medicine that ignores the transcendent therefore will be incomplete. I suggest that many of the contemporary controversies in medical ethics result from confused attempts to solve subjective, universal, and infinite problems through exclusively objective, particular, and finite means.

Pain and Suffering

A discussion of the meaning of medicine most properly begins with a discussion of pain and suffering. Although the two terms often are used synonymously, suffering and pain are different. Even though pain is intimately related to the psychological milieu in which it is experienced, it is fundamentally a biological phenomenon. The physiological basis of pain is something human beings share with other organisms. Excitation of certain neurons causes reflexive reactions (such as the removal of one's hand from a hot stove), as well as conscious, voluntary reactions (such as when one stops running upon feeling a cramp in the thigh).

The psychological milieu in which the experience of pain is most fully developed and complex is in humans, but other forms of animal life also have limited psychological experiences of pain. Even at the cellular level of organization, for example, pain is modified by previous experience. Research into the "modulation" phenomenon seems to indicate that pain receptor cells adjust their thresholds in reaction to signals from surrounding cells.[1] This finding has clinical significance. For example, the pain thresholds of various cultural groups appear to differ.[2] Depressed patients appear to experience more intense pain than nondepressed patients, even when their levels of illness and injury are the same.[3]

Not all pain causes suffering, however, and not all suffering is caused by pain. As Pope John Paul II once wrote, suffering is "something which is still wider than sickness, more complex and at the same time still more deeply rooted in humanity itself."[4] An athlete can experience pain in training but would not be said to suffer. A couple experiencing marital difficulties might suffer greatly, yet not be sick or experience pain. Nevertheless, the paradigmatic experiences of human suffering are experienced in the context of pain and sickness. The goals of the art and science of medicine are directed precisely toward these experiences. To understand medicine, one must understand suffering.

Only persons can suffer.[5] Even though the pain of animals is close to that of human beings, "nevertheless what we express by the word suffering seems to be particularly essential" to the nature of human beings.[6] Thus, an adequate philosophical anthropology (or understanding of the human person) would seem necessary to have an adequate understanding of suffering and, therefore, to understand medicine.[7] Although the development of a complete philosophical or theological anthropology is beyond the scope of this book, we might regard the work of Karl Rahner as an appropriate starting point.[8] Exploration of the relationship between the problem of suffering and the more general problem of evil also is beyond the scope of this book, although it is a vital part of the theology of suffering.[9]

For the limited points I want to make here, however, I need only take note of two characteristics of persons. First, the notion of a person as a being-in-relationship to others (i.e., family, friends, community, and culture) seems important if one is to understand the problem of the conscious suffering of a competent adult human being.[10] Second, the transcendent dimension of the human person also is critical to an understanding of suffering.[11] Such elements help to fill in the outlines left by Paul Ramsey when he called for a theory of medicine that would treat all patients as persons.[12]

As I have suggested elsewhere, suffering can be defined as an experience that makes explicit a person's actual finitude.[13] This experience need not be limited to physical pain or the threat of physical pain. Suffering can come about when persons confront their finitude—physically, morally, socially, or intellectually. Such a definition of suffering, though not theological, seems adequate to cover the requirements of a theological definition as well.[14]

In the context of the medical care of a conscious, competent, adult human being, suffering can be understood as a *meaning* a person assigns to his or her own experience of bodily finitude through sickness and pain. Ultimately, the meaning of all suffering is death. Suffering is a premonition of the ultimate dissolution of one's own person. Sickness and pain are the foretaste of death, which threatens to sunder the integrity of the embodied person. Behind every twinge of pain, beneath every wave of nausea, and within every drop of blood, the shadow of death is lurking. As Aquinas wrote, "Sickness is the privation of health, not that it removes health entirely, but that it is an approach to the whole losing of health, which is realized in death."[15] Medicine, as a professional enterprise, confronts the suffering brought on by sickness and pain. Such suffering occurs in a context shaped by all other forms of suffering— including rejection and loneliness, which are forms of distress brought about by apprehending one's finitude as a being-in-relationship: another form of death. Medicine confronts suffering under the shadow of death. A theory of medicine that addresses only sickness and pain, but not suffering, is inadequate.[16]

Subjectivity and Objectivity

Sickness always has deep, subjective, personal significance. As Soko-lowski has observed, the need for medical care is not like the need for automobile repairs or a haircut. "The medical [need] is special not because my body is at issue, but because *I* am at issue."[17] It is always an *I* who suffers, who goes to the doctor.

The subjective experience of sickness is what the medical profession traditionally has called a symptom. The most general and basic of all symptoms is expressed succinctly when a patient says, "I just don't feel *myself* today." Symptoms are distinguished from signs. Signs are what others (i.e., doctors and nurses) observe as the effects of sickness. Some symptoms cannot be observed and can only be reported—for example, the symptom of seeing yellow halos around lights. Some signs can be observed directly only by others and cannot be experienced subjectively or even observed of oneself directly, such as an asymptomatic change in the surface of the retina. Often, signs and symptoms are intrinsically linked. The same phenomenon can have two sides: It can be experienced as a symptom and observed as a sign. For example, a patient may experience the *symptom* of feeling hot. If a doctor observes this patient, the doctor may note that the patient has, among other *signs*, a fever. It is always a symptom, however, that leads a patient to seek medical attention—and symptoms are absolutely subjective.

Sympathy, Empathy, and Compassion

The definitions of these related words are contested. Because they are critical to any account of spirituality and health care, however, I offer my own analysis, using my own stipulative (but evocative) definitions.

Sickness arises in the pure subjectivity of persons. Yet persons are beings-in-relationship. Thus, the sickness and suffering of one person may move another person to deep sympathy. Sympathy connotes an experience of one's own suffering in the understanding that another suffers. Yet sympathy is not an understanding *of* the suffering of the other. Sympathy meets the subjectivity of another's suffering with one's own subjectivity. Sympathy says, "I feel bad because you feel bad." Thus, sympathy has no objective meaning. Sympathy alone is inadequate to the needs of sick persons because the sick person demands that his or her subjective state be verified, recognized, and accepted as objectively true.

An alternative response to the suffering of another is empathy. Empathy has a different connotation and meets the suffering of another on a deeper level of interpersonal experience. Empathy is an attempt to understand the suffering actually experienced by another—to *know* the suffering of another. Yet one must acknowledge that, no matter how much one cares, one can never completely understand the suffering another experiences. Perfect empathy is impossible, if only because one is not (and cannot ever become) the other. One cannot fully objectively know the subjectivity of another's suffering. Thus, empathy is not enough for the sick person. It is merely an attempt by one subjectivity to grasp another. It lacks the objectivity that sick persons require.

Beyond empathy, however, is the way of compassion. Compassion is a third and deeper response to the suffering of another.[18] Compassion is the mandate of the gospel, a central message of the Parable of the Good Samaritan (Luke 10:25–37). St. Bonaventure wrote that the Samaritan "poured into the wounds of that half-dead wanderer the wine of fervent zeal and the oil of compassion."[19] Compassion is the stuff of healing. Compassion demands recognition and response. Compassion touches the subjective core of the person who suffers, yet the ground of compassion is the objectivity that is inseparable from every suffering person's experience—namely, that although suffering is inherently subjective, all persons, as an objective fact, suffer. Each human suffers and has a need for understanding and care, and each shares in the persistent human question of the meaning of suffering. Compassion is an objective, concrete response to the subjective needs of the one who suffers. The offer of a cup of herbal tea to soothe a sick stomach means that the symptom is concrete, objective, and real because of the shared faith that it can be relieved by concrete, objective, and real actions. True compassion simultaneously addresses the physical, interpersonal, moral, and intellectual finitude of the whole person, binding the wounds and expressing genuine concern. Compassion requires that the compassionate "other" should stop and recognize the suffering of a fellow traveler who lies wounded on the side of the road—not out of curiosity but out of availability, and with a disposition of the heart that motivates one to help. Ultimately, compassion requires one to give of oneself.[20] Compassion is dialectically synthetic, making something new out of the subjective and objective, the finite and infinite, the particular and universal moments that erupt in the event of an individual's sickness. The sick person's need is for compassion.

The Dialectic of the Unwell

Having discussed pain and suffering and compassion in a general way, I now discuss the phenomenology of medicine more specifically. I distinguish four stages in the phenomenological development of the awareness of being unwell, showing how each stage gives rise to new dialectically opposed moments that ultimately can only be resolved by a spiritual understanding of the phenomenon of illness. By being *unwell* I mean a person's subjective awareness of an alteration in the physical status quo. By *sickness* I mean a person's own subjective recognition of the objective element in the awareness that one is unwell. By *illness* I mean the recognition of one person's sickness by a nonprofessional other. Finally, by *disease* I mean the socially sanctioned professional diagnosis given to the illness.

I offer an extended interpretation of the unfolding of this dialectic in human history, focusing particularly on the dialectic of disease and the history of medicine. These stages ought not be considered strictly chronological, however, with respect to the personal experience of individuals. They operate across the temporal unfolding of unwellness in the shared understanding of patients and healers in individual episodes down through the ages. Nor are these stages meant to be mutually exclusive. They are dialectically inclusive. One and the same person is initially unwell, ultimately decides that he or she feels sick, is noted by a relative to be ill, and goes to the doctor for diagnosis and treatment of a disease.

Unwellness

Homeostasis is a characteristic feature of biological organisms. Homeostasis means that organisms tend to maintain their integrity and balance relative to their environment. The environment, by contrast, tends to follow the law of entropy, toward undifferentiated randomness. Persons possess a consciousness that allows them to become aware of deviations from homeostasis. An alteration in homeostasis generally is the objective basis for the subjective perception that one is sick.[21]

For example, a rhinovirus might begin to disturb homeostasis by infecting the nasal mucosa of the throat, resulting in cell death, the release of inflammatory mediators, and swelling. The first awareness might be a sensation in the throat that is not quite painful. This sensation often occurs before the person is certain that he or she is sick; the person knows only that something is not right—all is not well. Thus, both objective and subjective moments synthetically characterize the state of unwellness. Objective alteration and subjective perception are both present in the unwell person. Objectively altered homeostasis does not become unwellness until it is subjectively perceived by the one whose homeostasis is disturbed.[22]

Sickness

The unwell person reflects on the subjective sense that something is wrong. The person may be unsure, however, and look for some objective sign to corroborate this subjective sense, such as seeing a rash, noting beads of sweat on the forehead, or looking in the mirror for spots on the tonsils. Such signs at first appear to provide the necessary objective verification of the subjective sense of unwellness: the harmonizing of the subjective sense that something is wrong with objective signs that the body has changed. The person thinks not just the undifferentiated thought "Something is wrong" but comes to the synthetic judgment "I am not myself. I am sick." The self that makes such a judgment is radically threatened by the implications of sickness. Self-validation seems inadequate in the face of the impending self-dissolution that is the *ultimate* meaning portended by the judgment, "I am not myself. I am sick." After all, even the rash is only a perception and therefore is invested with subjectivity. Is the perception correct? Has illness altered perception? Is the perception itself the illness (i.e., a hallucination)? The self-threatened-by-sickness has sought objectivity in the sign but does not know objectively whether the sign is really objective or abnormal. Moreover, discovery of a sign of illness does not assuage suffering. The apprehension that "I am not myself" is an apprehension of finitude. The self suffers. The self cannot be satisfied only with the judgment "I am sick."

Illness

Although the suffering sick person's experience begins as pure subjectivity, it must become objective for the suffering person's experience to be humanly actual and the sick person to become a patient. Suffering without objectification is intolerable to the human person. Self-validation is inadequate. One can become a patient (from the Latin, *patior*, to suffer) only when one's suffering has been objectively recognized. Unrecognized suffering is a more radical experience of one's finitude than the sickness itself that threatens bodily death.[23] No suffering is as profound as suffering alone. Solitary suffering is a state of total aloneness, abandonment, and dissolution. Hence the prospect of suffering and dying alone is terrifying. The subjective symptoms of sickness must be communicated to another for objective recognition. Signs of sickness must be recognized by another in confirmation of the symptoms. Until another recognizes that one is ill, one is not a patient.[24]

It is in illness that the subjectivity of pain and sickness becomes objective for another. Sociologists describe this phenomenon as social permission for the sick person to become a patient and assume "the sick role."[25] This phenomenon generally has its first unfolding in the context of family life. At its most primitive level, this is the moment in which the child first says to its mother, "I feel sick."[26] The mother, if she recognizes the child's suffering through the objective dimensions of the sickness (noting the warm forehead, the rash, the look in the eyes of the child, and the symptoms as communicated), takes the child close to her and whispers, "Don't worry. Everything is going to be okay." In so doing, she addresses the child's primitive terror, the fear of dissolution, the inchoate fear of death, by an act of recognition and prognostication. The child's suffering has an objective meaning, verified in the mother's recognition of the illness (fever and rash) and the prognosis ("With mother here, I will not die").

Infinity and Finitude

Even in this primitive first moment of illness—whether in the fifth century BCE or the twenty-first century CE—on becoming a patient with an illness and a prognosis, two sets of dialectically opposed moments immediately arise. In illness, the finite is opposed to the infinite and the particular is opposed to the universal. Illness represents a synthesis in which the subjectivity of sickness has been folded into the objectivity subtended by the confirmation others provide. This synthesis is unstable, however. These opposed moments are still in dialectical tension.

First, illness brings finitude and infinity into opposition. The finitude at stake is the finitude of the mortality that illness represents. The infinity at stake is the infinity of the need for healing, which really represents a need for immortality. The need for healing ultimately is an infinite need—a need to be free from the limitations that illness imposes, arising precisely in the reality of the limitations imposed by illness. Even if this illness passes, one knows that eventually there will be an illness that will not pass. Aware of one's own mortality, one cannot rationally expect one's ultimate need for healing to be fully met. Moreover, although the *need* for healing is necessarily infinite, medical technology is just as necessarily finite. Health care practitioners are finite. Patients are finite. Therefore, the need for healing is a need that stands opposed to its necessary failure. For example, a child eventually realizes that Mother has limited medical skills. Mother is mortal. Mother's prognosis that "everything will be okay" may turn out to be true in the short run, but as children grow up they realize that, in the long run, Mother's words are a lie. One day everything will not be okay. Each mature patient eventually realizes the reality of his or her own finitude. Something more than Mother is required. The synthesis represented by the stage of *illness* is inadequate to the needs of the suffering person.

Universality and Particularity

The stage of illness also brings the universal and particular moments of medicine into dialectical opposition. The need for healing is universal to the human condition. No death occurs except through an alteration in homeostasis—the unwellness in which all illness begins. The time interval between the altered homeostasis and death may be very short (e.g., a bullet wound to the head) or quite long (e.g., multiple sclerosis). Death and altered homeostasis are inextricably tied together, however, and universal to the human condition. *Sub specie aeternatis*, every person is a patient.

The universal need for healing stands dialectically opposed, however, to the absolute particularity of being unwell. The homeostasis of one individual is never disturbed in exactly the same way as that of another. No two persons experience sickness in the same way. The particular circumstances surrounding the sickness and the particularities of those who recognize the sickness as illness are always unique. Hence, the child eventually realizes that Mother also is particular. She cannot represent any of the universality of the need for healing. Her expertise is merely particular. It has no other basis than her own experience. It is directed only toward the particularity of her own children. Ultimately, Mother's efforts at healing must fail.

Disease

Therefore, the synthesis provided by the shared consciousness that characterizes the stage of illness inevitably breaks down. Verification of one's illness provided by a nonprofessional other (whether mother, father, spouse, or friend) is inadequate. Infinite need has been met with a merely finite response. Universal need has been met with a merely particular response. The intersubjectivity provided by the other has not provided the actual objectivity required to diagnose, to relieve suffering, and to heal. Mother's promises have failed. She is not a genuine healer.

The Witch Doctor

From the beginning of recorded history, then, ill persons have looked outside their families to others for help. These others must offer a socially mediated response to the predicament of illness that goes beyond the limits of family. The institution of the Witch Doctor, or tribal healer, stands as the first historical social mediation between all the dialectically opposed moments that illness represents. The Witch Doctor, shaman, or tribal healer brings the patient a universal healing otherness, which the universality of the patient's need requires. This universality is provided first and foremost by the gods—mediated by the Witch Doctor, on behalf of the tribe—and is brought to the particularity of the patient. In the Witch Doctor, medicine first became a social institution in human history.[27]

For the patient, the subjective and infinite need for healing is objectively met in the objectivity and finitude of the Witch Doctor—who, though particular, also is all of the universality of family, tribe, and divinity in his healing power. Not only is the subjective experience of sickness made objective by the Witch Doctor's recognition of the symptoms and signs of an actual diagnosis; not only is the fear of finitude and dissolution (which is suffering) mitigated by the Witch Doctor's prognostication. The Witch Doctor mediates the infinite power of healing in and through his own finitude, by an actual and particular act of healing. Thus, the Witch Doctor's healing is spiritual healing, incorporating the transcendent questions of the patient into a ritualized form of healing that answers these transcendent questions. The Witch Doctor also is the Universal Healing Other and the objectification of illness that the particular patient, in all the subjectivity of his or her suffering, requires. Simultaneously, the Witch Doctor brings the particular, finite, and objective healing that the Universal Patient, in his or her infinite need for healing, requires to be concretely healed. The herb is applied, and the patient recovers. The diagnosis and the treatment are supremely objective. The healing will of the gods brings an infinite subjectivity. The subjective and the objective, the universal and the particular, the finite and the infinite, are one synthetic act for the Witch Doctor. His patients are healed.

The initial moment of illness, in which the subjectivity of illness is made objective in the family, gives way to a greater subjective claim for infinite health and eternal life, which can be met only by a social institution—the Witch Doctor—folding the subjectivity of illness into the objectivity of *disease* and bringing healing on behalf of god and tribe. Healing by the Witch Doctor therefore is invested in ritual and prayer—religious images that convey the spiritual truth of healing. The Witch Doctor's training involves religious rituals of preparation, often at personal peril. The Witch Doctor exercises great social and political power in the tribe because each member knows that he or she will one day need him. The Witch Doctor stands *between* the tribe and the member, as well as *for* the tribe and for each member. For the tribe and all its members, the Witch Doctor is universal healing particularly mediated and infinite need circumscribed by his own finitude.

Medicine as Craft

The institution of the tribal healer has been all but swept away by the stream of Western history. As the age of reason in medicine dawned in ancient Greece, the first crack appeared in the relationship between medicine and religion. The inefficacy of the tribal healer, once hidden behind the veil of religion, was exposed by Greek reason. As an actual, concrete healer, the traditional religious practitioner was a naked failure. His patients often did not recover. All of them eventually died. Rational Greek medicine promised the efficacy of a medical practice based on empirical knowledge, not an invocation of the gods. In the new

Greek medicine, healing was based on observation and reasoning by the physician. As this rational approach to medicine developed and the direct role of religion in healing came to be regarded as superstition, the pre-Hippocratic Greek physician gradually assumed the role of craftsman. Patient and physician became two individuals with the merely particular concerns of craftsman and customer. The synthesis provided by religious healing had been all but annihilated.[28]

These first embryonic expressions of reason in medicine took the form of mere craft-reasoning by the pre-Hippocratic physician. The physician became a craftsman, concretely concerned in his own particularity with the concrete and merely particular needs of a particular patient and that patient's disease. The practice of the medical *techne* became a mere occupation, a means of earning a living. The physician became not a religious figure but a craftsman selling his wares, like anyone else in the marketplace. Yet because the physician's diagnosis and treatment were based on reason (even if only craft-reasoning), his empirical efficacy triumphally superseded the incantations of the tribal healer. The physician's practice made more sense, and it worked better.

Medicine as a Profession

Such a situation could not long remain tolerable, however, for the physician or for the patient. The universality inherent in the fact that all persons, subjectively, need healing required a universality in the healing process. The pre-Hippocratic Greek physician, aware of the universality in the power of healing and reason, could not long tolerate the restrictions placed on his freedom by the concrete particularity of medicine practiced as a mere occupation. The Hippocratic Oath—and with it the concept of medicine as a profession—offered a solution. With the oath, medicine became for the first time a profession.

I address the topic of oaths in greater detail in chapter 6. Here, however, I note that in the oath, as an act of profession, a public act of self-dedication by the healer, the universal moment in medicine was restored.[29] The gods were not divorced from medicine because of reason, but the reason of medicine was made actual *through* a religious act.

In the actuality of the spoken words of the physician, who swore the oath by invoking the names of the gods, and in the actuality of the physician's adherence to the moral content of the oath, the transcendent had a role in medicine. In the profession—which the physician entered only through the oath—the particularity of the physician as a mere medical craftsman was integrated into the universality of a fellowship of practitioners who formed a brotherhood, educating each other and the coming generations of physicians. In Hippocratic medicine, the particular empirical knowledge of the individual physician as a craftsman was integrated into the universal knowledge of a profession—one that practiced rational medicine as a universal art, bound by an oath to the gods.

The essential particularity of the practice of medicine can never be ignored, however, and the Hippocratic physicians fully realized the inseparability of the universal and the particular moments of their enterprise. Medicine is an art that is practiced in particular ways by particular clinicians on behalf of particular patients. Nonetheless, this healing art is informed by a science that is oriented to universals. Medicine ministers to a universal need for healing, one particular person at a time. This is what it means to say that medicine is both a science and an art. The Hippocratic Oath implicitly expressed the conviction that the synthesis of the science and art of medicine can be achieved only through an invocation of the transcendent.

The oath was not sworn only before other doctors. A professional brotherhood ultimately is just a finite sum of particular doctors. The oath was sworn before the gods. The particular prognostications and purgatives of the Hippocratic physician actualized the healing of the gods. The universality inherent in the reason of rational Greek medicine informed each professional act for each particular patient. The patient's particularity itself became subsumed in the Hippocratic-professional synthesis. The patient became idealized by the profession, whose members swore by the gods to serve the patient under a code of behavior. This code, which was universal to the profession, became the actual and concrete ethical life lived and practiced by physicians. Religion, as ethical life, again came to play a decisive role in medicine. A sense of duty to the patient, and even sacrifice, became the equivalent of the shamanistic rites of initiation by which the doctor was sanctioned by society to care for sick persons. The infinite needs of the patient were now met in the finitude of the Hippocratic physician who mediated the infinite healing of the gods, made concrete in the rationality of medicine, for the finite patient, subsumed under the oath.

Covenant

As I discuss in chapter 4, in ancient Judaism healing and divinity were so deeply intertwined that any human attempts to heal were considered presumptuous and scandalous forays into the exclusive province of the deity. Yet while the Hellenized Hebrews struggled to prevent undue pagan influence, nonetheless they were anxious to reap all permissible benefits from advanced Greek medicine. Gradually, Jewish religious authorities loosened their long-standing prohibitions on the practice of medicine and began to allow this new rational healing to be practiced among Jews. They did this by interpreting rational Greek medicine as a gift from the God of Abraham, not from Apollo, and by making the doctor the mediator of God's covenant with the Chosen People in the domain of healing. Rational medicine could be regarded as a gift from Yahweh, divorced from the abominations of pagan healing rituals. Because healing could come only from the Lord, Ben Sira concluded that it was the Lord who "gave skill to human beings that he might be glorified in his mighty works. By them the physician heals and takes away pain" (Sir. 38:6–7). God's infinite healing was to be mediated through the rational finitude of the professional practice of medicine. The covenant between the people and Yahweh, the true source of healing, informed and energized a covenant between the doctor and the patient. This "covenant within a covenant" was—in accord with the knowledge of its era—truly spiritual and truly scientific.

Technological Medicine

The synthesis forged by the Hellenized Hebrews was essentially the same as the synthesis eventually adopted by European Christians and

Jews.[30] In Christianity, sick persons were regarded as having a truly "preferential" position in society. By the time of the early Middle Ages, most European physicians were either priests or monks, who continued, in a sense, the healing ministry of Christ. The concept of a covenant between doctor and patient, set within the larger covenant between God and God's people, implicitly governed the European understanding of medicine for centuries. The paradoxes inherent in medicine were subsumed in this grand Judeo-Christian synthesis.

Historical developments over the past several centuries have radically undermined this synthesis, however. The birth of Foucault's clinic brought profound challenges for the Judeo-Christian synthesis. For several centuries after the Enlightenment, a humanistic sense of professionalism served many physicians and patients as an alternative to the Judeo-Christian model. Practitioners of Enlightenment medicine could still point to the profession as a brotherhood and a service to humanity. Although stripped of any explicit religious meaning and not universal or infinite in its scope, this humanistic sense of professionalism nonetheless did point beyond the particular finitude of the individual doctor-patient encounter to something bigger. The birth of the modern scientific clinic changed all this, however.

Now, at the beginning of the twenty-first century, the erosive currents of history have worn away even this humanistic-professional model. As a result, contemporary Western medicine finds itself on the verge of conceptual incoherence, pulled apart by multiple, apparently irreconcilable, dialectically opposed moments.

History of Medical Technology

The role of religion probably faded faster in medicine than in other aspects of Western culture. The old medicine, practiced even into the eighteenth and nineteenth centuries by the kindly bedside professional who shared a basic Judeo-Christian tradition with his patient and understood practice as a covenant, eventually proved nearly as inefficacious as the practices of the Witch Doctor. Leeches cured no one.

Castor oil and enemas helped only a few. When various preparations—such as digitalis leaf for dropsy—did seem to work, the means by which healing occurred were not understood. It became clear that the "rational medicine" of the seventeenth century and before had almost no rational treatments—only serendipitous discoveries that almost anyone could have made without the help of any professional knowledge. From Moliere to Shaw, ridicule was justly leveled against the profession.

Scientific medicine began to make a difference, however, especially in the twentieth century. Foucault's clinic exercised its dominion. Infectious diseases came to be understood through the development of germ theory, and some were prevented or even cured. Insulin was discovered in the 1920s and saved the lives of countless diabetics. Vaccines and antisera were introduced before World War II. During and after the war, antibiotics were introduced. Suddenly pneumonia, syphilis, endocarditis, and countless other previously lethal diseases were cured through scientific medicine. More recently, advances unimaginable only a few decades ago have begun to occur in rapid succession. Imaging techniques such as computerized axial tomography (CAT) scanners, surgical techniques such as vascular bypass and transplantation, and the cure of some cancers through chemotherapy are just a few examples. With the dawning of the age of molecular medicine, technology seems to hold even greater promises. The potential has appeared infinite to many observers. There has been no need to invoke any gods. Human science, not divine knowledge, has provided these cures. Religion has been relegated to quackery and superstition and feeble attempts at cure that have no objective efficacy. Professionalism has replaced covenant, and science has replaced art. Yet now the very concept of medicine as scientific professionalism is on the brink of falling apart.

Technology also has forced an increasing degree of specialization and scientific, objective detachment on the part of practitioners. No practitioner can be master of all the knowledge and all the techniques. Physicians increasingly have become masters of particular, objective domains. Patients have become the loci of these objective domains.

Antinomies of the Medical-Industrial Complex

The success of technology also has led to increasing complexity in the economic, political, and social relationships of medical practice. Arnold Relman has dubbed this phenomenon the "medical-industrial complex."[31] The monetary cost of providing such medicine has risen dramatically. Increasingly, in an effort to control these costs through competition, the physician has been encouraged to practice either as an individual entrepreneur or as the employee of very large-scale entrepreneurial ventures.

These developments have resulted in a state in which the antinomies of medicine are now acutely, painfully, and ominously obvious. To date, however, understanding of how these conflicts have arisen has been explained in terms of a long-standing argument between liberalism and libertarianism—two schools of thought that tend to share the same basic assumptions of possessive individualism.[32] Interpretations such as the one I am presenting have not been aired in this milieu. I assume, however, that the ultimate needs of the patient remain the same now as ever.

The roots of the conflicted state of contemporary medicine lie largely in the fact that contemporary medicine and contemporary society have failed to address these ultimate needs and have broken the medical enterprise apart into the polarities of all its dialectical moments. Technological developments in medicine have not been synthetically integrated into a theory of medicine that is adequate to the needs of human persons at the dawn of the twenty-first century. Foucault's clinic is concerned exclusively with the inanimate substrates of chemistry and electricity. In other words, that clinic is dead.

The promise of technology continues to persist as the illusion of an infinite response to the infinite needs of patients. Western society is now beginning to face the reality, however, that technology is finite.

Patients' needs for healing are as infinite as ever. Technology once appeared capable of curing every disease and giving the gift of eternal health. Physicians have deluded themselves and others (perhaps through a grand exercise in the denial of death) into almost believing that this is true.[33] They have seen no need to call on any god for the infinite term in medical practice. Their power has come from science.

Medical consumerism is another sign of this misguided understanding. Patients now shop in an indefinite, ongoing search for immortality and are never satisfied by what they consume. The eventual death of the patient has come to be regarded as a failure and perhaps even a recoverable grievance. Because medicine, of course, is finite, the best medicine could possibly hope to offer patients (and medicine is far from this capability) would be indefinite ongoingness, but never the true infinity of immortality. Technology cannot transcend the finite. The story of technological medicine is the story of the Sibyl of Cumae—who, having been granted her request for "eternal life" but not having received the gift of eternal youth, was left wandering, shriveled, carried about in a jar, asking for death.[34] This story is played out daily in intensive care units throughout this country. Technological progress is finite.[35] The need for healing remains infinite.

The physician as professional is a universal figure. The physician as specialist and entrepreneur is particular. The late twentieth century witnessed the "deprofessionalization" of medical practice, motivated by a desire for specialized technological skills and by an overwrought egalitarianism that misconstrued professionalism as elitism. Yet the need for medicine remains universal to the human condition. The healers who will serve the needs of sick persons must have a truly universal term to heal in a full and complete fashion. The fragmentation that has resulted from increasingly specialized and entrepreneurial practice (medicine practiced only in the self-interest of the practitioners) is a stark denial of the universal term of medicine. For a variety of reasons, many medical schools have now dispensed with the Oath of Hippocrates, replacing it with vague statements designed to be inoffensive to everyone and consequently having meaning to no one.[36] Moreover, medical specialization has progressed to the point where some observers are now suggesting that the aggregate of subspecialties and sub-subspecialties no longer really constitutes a single profession. The universal need for healing is being met today by healers who see themselves and others as increasingly particular.

Technological medicine has focused almost exclusively on the objective elements in disease. This focus has been responsible for its remarkable success. Technological medicine has reached a point, however, where *only* the objectivity of the disease and its elimination are of importance. Suffering often is ignored and unrecognized. Medicine increasingly has lost the subjective term that compassion demands. Diseases are cured, but persons are not healed. Medicine has failed to recognize the subjectivity of suffering. As a result, the more successful medicine has become in providing cures, the less satisfied patients have become.

Medical Consumerism

Once the doctor was no longer regarded as a professional whose rational practice brought divinely mediated healing, medicine could not address the patient's infinite needs. This phenomenon partially explains the desperate attempts of so many patients to fill this need through ceaseless consumption of medical resources in an impossible quest to ward off illness and death. The medical profession itself has helped to foster these consumptive appetites and generated false hopes. The appetites of patients, in turn, have fed the self-interest of physicians who self-identify as entrepreneurs. Having largely abandoned their truly professional commitment to self-effacement and serving the needs of their patients first, physicians also have become dissatisfied, trapped in the particularity of medicine practiced as mere occupation.[37] Without a transcendent term, every action taken for every patient becomes merely determinate, particular, trivial, and ultimately doomed to failure. For many physicians, making money has become an attempt to fill this void through continual accumulation of particular and finite fees that can never satisfy the ultimate term of the physician's own stated will to heal. The physician is set against the patient, without meaningful relationship to the transcendent terms of profession, society, or religion.

Utilitarian Attempts to Control Demand

In recognition of the finitude of resources, many policy experts recently have proposed that the solution to the fiscal and ethical problems facing contemporary medicine lies in incorporating social utility into medical decision making by doctors and patients.[38] Doctors increasingly are urged to practice "population medicine" and to shift their emphasis from individual patients to improving the health of the entire population of patients under their care.[39] Unfortunately, this response is insufficient to the problems I have outlined.

First, social utility ultimately is finite, not infinite, and cannot meet the need for the truly infinite in medicine. A true common good is greater than the sum of its parts.[40] The common good of utilitarians is atomistic. It is nothing more than the sum of the interests of each individual, divided by their number. Second, in striving to be universal, utilitarianism ignores the particular; hence it also is inadequate for the needs of medicine. As Rawls has written, "Utilitarianism does not take seriously the distinction between persons."[41] The particularities of each person and each case are swept away by the utilitarian calculus. In striving for the objectivity of an "unseen spectator" who can coolly calculate the net ratio of utility to disutility for any proposal across the aggregate of society's members, utilitarianism ignores the subjective. The spectator of utilitarianism is not so much invisible as blind. If utilitarians try instead to judge suffering *subjectively*, allowing each individual to create his or her own utility scale, they face the insurmountable problem of incommensurability. There is no absolute anchoring value of suffering *objectively* shared by all people.[42] Subjective utility scales are incommensurable between persons. Intersubjectivity does not and cannot add up to objectivity. Thus, utilitarianism fails as a synthetic response to the disparate moments of the medical enterprise at the dawn of the twenty-first century.

Toward a Spiritual Scientific Medicine

The situation is not hopeless. Rebirth is possible. I suggest, boldly, that spirituality alone can provide the synthesis necessary for this rebirth. Spirituality can bring healing to health care. Although contemporary scientific medicine is extraordinarily efficacious, it is not infinitely efficacious. This acknowledgment is a point of reference. A spiritual-scientific medicine would be both practically efficacious in its scientific aspect and open to the transcendent dimensions of the patient as person in its spiritual aspect. What follows is a sketch of what shape this vision might take: a plan for a renewed covenant in medicine, at once scientific and spirit-filled.

A New Medical Covenant

If one reads the signs of the times through faith (e.g., Luke 12:56), nothing could seem more critical to health care than the need for a new medical covenant. The synthesis that the Witch Doctor represented in antiquity eventually was superseded by the Judeo-Christian interpretation of rational medicine practiced as a covenant. Today, therefore, the ascendancy of technological medicine and the consequent dissipation of the meaning of humanistic-professional medicine will require a new synthesis. A new spiritual interpretation of health care might be just that synthesis.

There will be no technological "quick fix" for the problems that beset contemporary medicine—the kind of solution so desperately sought by technocrats. What is required seems to be no less than a form of conversion for patients and health care practitioners: their rediscovery of the spiritual meaning of sickness, suffering, and health care.

Particular and Transcendent

Medicine must remain scientific. Its efficacy depends on science, and science is part of its universal term. Yet the science of medicine cannot be confused with technology. The science of medicine must be studied in the context of the universality of a profession dedicated to the service of bodily suffering that is universal to the human condition. In the universality of a profession, medicine itself, not just the particular doctor, heals the patient. Medical science conceived as entrepreneurship is not adequate. It fails to meet fully the universality that medical practice requires.

Medicine is not sometimes an art and sometimes a science. It is always simultaneously both art and science. Individual maladies afflict whole persons. Ironically, the apparent hyperspecialization of molecular genetics may provide the first steps toward acquiring such an understanding.[43] The differences among subspecialists working at the molecular level are beginning to dissolve. The DNA in a human brain cell, a human liver cell, and a human bone cell is the same. Physician-scientists trained as oncologists conducting research in the molecular biology of cancer could become rheumatologists tomorrow. As molecular medicine helps to reconstitute a sense of the unity of the body, finding the universality inherent in the particularity of the single gene, perhaps the profession will soon recover a sense of the whole person and recognize the synthetic unity of medicine as an art and a science, as a way to serve the universal human condition of suffering as well as a way to make a living.

In recognition of the universality of the need for healing, a profession and society informed by such a consciousness would recognize the duty to provide care for each particular person who has that need. Medicine might then take the necessary steps toward reconstituting itself as a profession. If medicine is to be a profession, in the fullest sense of the word, it must recognize that it can transcend the limits of its own particularity only if all its particular members practice in a spirit of faith, hope, and love.

Such a medical science also would then be understood again as a *covenant* between doctors and patients, requiring that medical investigation be conducted as a service, with trustworthiness and fidelity. Physician scientists would not own stock in the companies that manufacture the drugs they are investigating; they would not engage in scientific fraud for the sake of career advancement; and they would not patent and claim to own sequences of human chromosomal anatomy as personal intellectual property.

Objective and Transcendent

Medicine must remain objective. It must be objective to recognize disease. It must be objective to remain efficacious. Yet medicine also must recognize the suffering of sick persons. In other words, medicine must be compassionate. It must objectify the subjective suffering of sick persons if its efficacy is to be more than superficial. Moreover, that recognition must move the health care practitioner to concrete, objective acts of healing. Care for sick persons is the most *corporal* of the works of mercy. The subjective needs of sick persons must be met through this corporeality.

This understanding is the physician's new covenant. It would demand, for example, spending more time with patients, not less; explaining more, listening more, and palpating with subjective concern as well as objective interest. Then no one would propose to reform health care by forcing patient visits into shorter and "more efficient" time slots. For the Christian physician, for instance, medicine might be practiced in the infinite subjectivity of the person of Jesus—who Christians believe recognizes all human suffering and saves the world by sharing in that suffering (Luke 4:23).

Finite and Transcendent

Medicine will remain finite. Professionals and patients must realize that even progress is not infinite. Medicine does not grant immortality. Yet because the needs of the sick are infinite, the entire medical enterprise is a failure unless it can incorporate the infinite into its praxis. Utility is merely finite. God is infinite. Thus, healing acts performed in the name of God can incorporate the infinity of the divine into diagnosis and treatment and meet the infinite needs of patients. Health care professionals who do not believe in God will be required to seek out some other source of transcendence—nature, or humanity, or the good, or something else that transcends patients, practitioners, and their professions—if they are to meet their own transcendent needs or those of their patients.

Practitioners and patients who understand this need for transcendence will share in a new medical covenant. They will arrive together, for example, at a recognition of the time when each patient's journey with illness has reached the limits of medical knowledge. The vain belief that immortality can be purchased from the medical profession on a fee-for-service basis will die its own natural death only when both doctor and patient are filled with an infinite hope that transcends the limits of technology and mortality.

Conclusion

Under this new medical covenant, a spiritual-scientific practitioner would affirm that the transcendent is made manifest at the edge of the surgeon's knife, at the tips of the palpating fingers of the pediatrician, in the firm handshake of the internist, in the birth of the child whose unwed mother has AIDS, in the tears of the woman who feels a hard lump in her one remaining breast, and in the vacant stare of the elderly man with dementia. A spiritual-scientific practitioner would affirm that the transcendent is there when disease and suffering are recognized together, when the hand that performs the spinal tap distills compassion into the needle's point—the objectivity of science with the subjectivity of God's healing will; the particularity of the case at hand with the universality of a profession under oath; the finitude of the moment and the infinity of a life lived in the service of love. Thus might the clinic be reborn.

Notes

1. Kathleen M. Foley and Ehud Arbit, "Management of Cancer Pain," in *Cancer: Principles and Practice*, 3rd ed., ed. Vincent T. DeVita, Samuel Hellman, and Steven A. Rosenberg (Philadelphia: J. B. Lippincott, 1989) , 2064–87.

2. H. P. Greenwald, "Interethnic Differences in Pain Perception," *Pain* 44 (1991): 157–63; R. Moore, M. L. Miller, P. Weinstein, S. F. Dworkin, and H. H. Liou, "Cultural Perceptions of Pain and Pain Coping among Patients and Dentists," *Community Dental and Oral Epidemiology* 14 (1986): 327–33;. M. Zborowski, "Cultural Components in Response to Pain," *Journal of Social Issues* 8 (1952): 15–35.

3. P. A. Parmelee, I. R. Katz, and M. P. Lawton, "The Relation of Pain to Depression among Institutionalized Aged," *Journal of Gerontology* 46 (1991): P15–21; J. A. Haythornthwaite, W. J. Sieber, and R. D. Kerns, "Depression and the Chronic Pain Experience," *Pain* 46 (1991): 177–84.

4. John Paul II, 1984, "*Salvifici Doloris*" (apostolic letter), *Origins* 13, no. 37 (February 23, 1984): 609–24.

5. Eric Cassell, "The Nature of Suffering and the Goals of Medicine," *New England Journal of Medicine* 306 (1982): 639–45.

6. John Paul II, "*Salvifici Doloris.*"

7. Klaus Demmer, "Theological Argument and Hermeneutics in Bioethics," in *Catholic Perspectives on Medical Morals*, ed. Edmund D. Pellegrino et al. (Amsterdam: Kluwer Academic Publishers, 1989), 103–22.

8. See, e.g., Karl Rahner, *Theology, Anthropology, Christology*, vol. 13 of *Theological Investigations*, trans. David Bourke (New York: Seabury, 1975); see also Karl Rahner, "Man (anthropology) III – theological," in *Sacramentum Mundi*, vol. 3, ed. Karl Rahner New York: Herder and Herder, 1969), 365–70.

9. John Paul II, "*Salvifici Doloris.*"

10. Cassell, "The Nature of Suffering and the Goals of Medicine." Note that some of the features Cassell associates with personhood—such as personality, memory, action, and concern about the future—are somewhat functional and, if taken as necessary features, risk excluding certain marginalized individuals from the community of persons. For this reason, I have chosen to exclude these other features from the list of features of persons and discuss only the paradigmatic case of the competent, conscious, adult human being. I do not address many related and very interesting questions, such as whether an individual in a state of permanent unconsciousness can in any sense be said to personally suffer.

11. John Paul II, "*Salvifici Doloris.*"

12. Paul Ramsey, *The Patient as Person* (New Haven, Conn.: Yale University Press, 1970).

13. Daniel P. Sulmasy, "Finitude, Freedom, and Suffering," in *Pain Seeking Understanding: Suffering, Medicine, and Faith*, ed. Mark J. Hanson and Margaret Mohrman (Cleveland: Pilgrim Press, 1999), 83–102.

14. John Paul II, "*Salvifici Doloris.*"

15. Thomas Aquinas, *Summa Theologica* I-II, q.18, a.8, ad. 1, in *Treatise on Happiness*, trans. John A. Osterle (Notre Dame, Ind.: University of Notre Dame Press, 1983), 171.

16. Cassell, "The Nature of Suffering and the Goals of Medicine."

17. Robert Sokolowski, "The Art and Science of Medicine," in *Catholic Perspectives on Medical Morals*, ed. Edmund D. Pellegrino et al. (Amsterdam: Kluwer Academic Publishers, 1989), 263–75.

18. See the account of suffering and compassion in Warren T. Reich, "Speaking of Suffering," *Soundings* 72 (1989): 83–108.

19. St. Bonaventure, *De sex alis seraphim*, trans. Sabinus Mollitor (St. Louis: B. Herder, 1920), 30.

20. John Paul II, "*Salvifici Doloris.*"

21. Edmond A. Murphy, "The Diagnostic Process, the Diagnosis, and Homeostasis," *Theoretical Medicine* 9 (1988): 151–66.

22. For some diseases, such as hypertension, there is no immediate awareness of an alteration in homeostasis (i.e., the disease is "asymptomatic"). In such cases, the immediate stages of unwellness, illness, and sickness are bypassed. Awareness of altered homeostasis comes only through the objective findings of a professional. Yet it can have the same meaning. For example, the "asymptomatic" hypertensive may begin to lose more work days after becoming aware of the disease. Similarly, the knowledge that one has an asymptomatic heart murmur can result in a behavioral response known as the "cardiac cripple."

23. Eric J. Cassell, "Recognizing Suffering," *Hastings Center Report* 21, no. 3 (May–June 1991): 24–31.

24. The somatization disorder (formerly hypochondriasis) is a disease in which the person has symptoms but no signs. Although the person misrepresents these symptoms as physical even though the physician recognizes the actual source as psychological, the physician nevertheless must objectively recognize the suffering of the subject if the person is to become a patient and not a "crock." In the absence of objective recognition of his or her suffering, the person will find the physician's judgment, "There is nothing wrong with you," completely intolerable and will seek another physician until he or she finds one who will mistakenly accept the symptoms as physical and thereby recognize the suffering. The only way to stop such a cycle and help such a person is to objectively recognize the suffering without validating the actual symptoms. In this way, the person becomes an actual patient.

25. Talcott Parsons, "The Sick Role," in *Patients, Physicians, and Illness*, 2nd ed., ed. E. G. Jaco (New York: Free Press, 1970), 101–27.

26. See William F. May, *The Physician's Covenant: Images of the Healer in Medical Ethics,* 2nd ed. (Lexington, Ky.: Westminster John Knox Press, 2000). The various relationships described in this chapter, corresponding to various levels of understanding between patients and other persons, share an interesting homology with the models of the doctor–patient relationship May describes. May's method was largely metaphorical, whereas mine is historical and dialectical, but a similar spectrum of descriptions arises in both methods. The difference is that I do not see these models of the doctor–patient relationship as *competing* but as necessary stages in a dialectical process in which each stage is somehow incorporated into the succeeding stage. All these stages persist in the relationships of patients with other people, as well as with physicians. Hence, sick persons still turn to mother or spouse for initial objectification of symptoms, and many persons will seek the healing of Western medicine and the healing of religious leaders simultaneously.

27. Mircea Eliade, *Shamanism* (New York: Pantheon, 1964); M. Gelfand, *Witch Doctor* (London: Harvill Press, 1964).

28. Darrel W. Amundsen and Gary B. Ferngren, "Evolution of the Patient-Physician Relationship: Antiquity through the Renaissance," in *The Clinical Encounter,* ed. Earl E. Shelp (Dordrecht, The Netherlands: D. Reidel, 1983), 3–46.

29. Edmund D. Pellegrino, "Toward a Reconstruction of Medical Morality: The Primacy of the Act of Profession and the Fact of Illness," *Journal of Medicine and Philosophy* 4 (1979): 32–56.

30. Amundsen and Ferngren, "Evolution of the Patient-Physician Relationship."

31. Arthur S. Relman, "The New Medical-Industrial Complex," *New England Journal of Medicine* 303 (1980): 963–70.

32. Norman Daniels, *Just Health Care* (London: Cambridge University Press, 1985); H. Tristram Engelhardt, *The Foundations of Bioethics* (New York: Oxford University Press, 1986), 336–74; C. B. MacPherson, *The Political Theory of Possessive Individualism: Hobbes to Locke* (New York: Oxford University Press, 1962).

33. See Ernst Becker, *The Denial of Death* (New York: Free Press, 1973).

34. Arbiter Petronius, *The Satyricon of Petronius*, trans. William Arrowsmith (Ann Arbor: University of Michigan Press, 1959), 47.

35. Daniel Callahan, "Death and the Research Imperative," *New England Journal of Medicine* 342 (2000): 654–56.

36. Daniel P. Sulmasy, "What Is an Oath and Why Should a Physician Swear One?" *Theoretical Medicine and Bioethics* 20 (1999): 329–46.

37. Jack Hadley, Jack and Jean M. Mitchell, "Effects of HMO Market Penetration on Physicians' Work Effort and Satisfaction," *Health Affairs* (Millwood) 16 (November–December 1997): 99–111.

38. See, for example, Paul T. Menzel, *Strong Medicine: The Ethical Rationing of Health Care* (New York: Oxford University Press, 1990); Henry J. Aaron and William B. Schwartz, *The Painful Prescription: Rationing Hospital Care* (Washington, D.C.: Brookings Institution Press, 1984); Daniel Callahan, *Setting Limits: Medical Goals in an Aging Society* (New York: Simon and Schuster, 1987).

39. Mark Hall and Robert A. Berenson, "Ethical Practice in Managed Care: A Dose of Realism," *Annals of Internal Medicine* 128 (1998): 395–402.

40. Daniel P. Sulmasy, "Four Basic Notions of the Common Good," *St. John's Law Review* 75 (2002): 303–10.

41. John Rawls, *A Theory of Justice* (Cambridge, Mass.: Harvard University Press, 1971), 27.

42. Jorgen Hilden, "The Non-Existence of Interpersonal Utility Scales: A Missing Link in Medical Decision Theory?" *Medical Decision Making* 5 (1985): 215–28.

43. Daniel P. Sulmasy, "The Fullness of Life: Integrating Patient Care, Teaching, and Research," *Health Progress* 74 (January 1993): 76–78.

6

Taking Physicians' Oaths Seriously

It is no secret that the medical profession today is deeply confused about its own identity. The historical forces I outline in chapter 5 have taken their toll. Medicine is radically threatened by external social forces, and its own internal logic of continuous scientific progress has set the profession on a course of self-deprofessionalization. Technological change has depersonalized the experience of practice as much for doctors as for patients. Specialization has balkanized the profession. Neuroradiologists wonder what they have in common with primary care pediatricians. The public has knocked doctors off their pedestals, and many doctors feel hurt. In the face of the "industrialization" of health care, many physicians feel more and more that they are simply cogs in a huge economic machine.

The Oath of Hippocrates traditionally has played a central role in defining the profession, and it has engendered much recent discussion and interest.[1] As I argue in chapter 5, the practice of oath-taking has played a significant role in the spiritual history of medicine, invoking transcendent witnesses and mediating the meaning of a profession as something that transcends individual practice. Many ethicists and commentators today, however, are arguing that physicians' oaths are nothing more than anachronistic formalities. No one pays attention to these oaths. Many practitioners disagree with the content of what is sworn. Hence, many of these commentators suggest doing away with the whole practice of asking physicians to swear oaths.[2]

The practice of oath-taking in general seems to have fallen on hard times. Recent events in American public life have called into question the importance and meaning of such oaths. Can anyone's oath, let alone a physician's oath, be taken seriously?

Oaths and Promises

It may help a bit to get clearer about what it means to swear an oath.[3] An oath is deeper than a simple promise. A promise is a declaration to do or not do some specific performance. There is nothing formal or necessarily public about a promise. A promise has moral binding force, of course. We ought to keep our promises. Kant says we should keep our promises because we could not make a failure to do so into a universal law without contradicting ourselves. In a world in which no one kept his or her word, intending not to keep one's word would be self-contradictory. In such a world, lying simply wouldn't work because lying depends on the expectation of truth.[4] W. D. Ross thinks that it is intuitively obvious that promises should be kept, at least as a *prima facie* principle.[5] If God forbids lying in the Ten Commandments, *a fortiori* all persons who feel obliged to keep those commandments should keep their promises.

Oaths share many of the features of promises. Oaths are more solemn, formal, infrequent, and general in content than promises, however. Oaths are addressed to a wide public audience and generally invoke a transcendent witness. They also seem to involve the person who swears them in a fundamental way. Persons who swear oaths are understood not just to have made temporary commitments to perform specified acts; the act of swearing an oath implies that the swearer is somehow changed as a person. For instance, the president of the United States takes an oath of office. This oath-taking is a very solemn, formal event. It happens only once every four years. The content is broad—to preserve, protect, and defend the Constitution of the United States. The oath is addressed primarily to the people of the United States, but in a very real sense it also is addressed to everyone in the world. The words "so help me God" invoke the heavens to provide the most transcendent witness possible. From that moment, until the end of the president's term or removal from office, the ordinary citizen who swears this oath becomes someone new—the president of the United States.

A vow is closer to an oath than a promise. Persons who marry profess public vows. Although the various apostolic societies in the Roman Catholic Church offer a wide variety of public and private vow-like bonds, persons who enter official, canonical religious life as monks, friars, or nuns take public vows.[6] Entering marriage or the religious life is an important undertaking, each requiring a serious, open-ended commitment intended to last a lifetime. Persons who take vows or oaths are *changed* because of the words they have spoken, the way in which they have spoken them, the setting in which the speaking has taken place, and the meaning and expectations assigned to that speaking.

Like a vow, an oath invokes a witness that transcends the audience to whom the words are addressed. In an oath, one is not simply making a promise as one individual to another. One is publicly declaring that the words one says are so significant that the event must be witnessed by something bigger than oneself and even bigger than the audience that hears the words. An oath is reserved for declarations serious enough to require a divine witness.

Physicians' Oaths

Physicians swear oaths upon graduation. They do more than make promises. The physicians' oath is a serious, binding commitment. It is a very public event. Those who swear it thereby make themselves accountable for their words. The most popular version used at American medical schools these days is the Modified Oath of Hippocrates.[7] This oath is a "pledge" to "lead my life and practice in uprightness and honor" and to work for the "good of the sick . . . to the utmost of my power." Graduates swear this oath by "whatever [they] hold most sacred." These words ought to be spoken in fear and in trembling. I suspect few students think about this oath, however, before they take the Medical College Admission Test.

Of course, physicians are not the only persons who swear oaths. Public officials and courtroom witnesses also take oaths, for example. All of these groups make serious, binding, public commitments. What do these disparate groups have in common? First, all three dedicate themselves to specific public service roles. Second, they commit themselves radically to honesty. Third, they all make themselves publicly accountable for these commitments.

If oath-taking is not to become a quaint relic of the ancient moral past, medical students will need to understand that the words of the oath have a serious moral purpose, and the persons to whom the oath is addressed (i.e., all their potential patients) will need to share this view. Therefore, an attempt to understand a bit more about the spiritual and moral purposes of a physician's oath seems appropriate.

The Physician's Oath as Spiritual Act

The swearing of the physician's oath has spiritual meaning. By the definition I have offered for spirituality, explicit invocation of the transcendent in the words of the oath automatically implies something spiritual. By whatever name a physician who swears the oath calls the transcendent, this name will point to the spiritual. The Hippocratic Oath invoked Apollo and Aesculapius. Contemporary Christian versions of the oath explicitly invoke God. Even the most secular versions use the phrase "whatever I hold most sacred." This phrase implies something beyond the mundane and the pedestrian. It implies something spiritual about the medical enterprise.

As the rite of passage into the profession, the oath also has a ritual character. However attenuated, the rite of swearing the oath as the formal entry into the profession has a religious flavor. Engineers and accountants do not undergo any sort of ritual of entry into their profession. They pursue noble and useful occupations, but they are not engaged in true professions, and they need not swear an oath to work.

The idea of a profession itself, as I argue in chapter 5, contains transcendent elements. To enter into a profession is to step beyond oneself into something greater that is not of one's own creation. The transcendence mediated by professionalism is critical in meeting the needs of sick persons and transforming the professional's self-understanding. Although the sense of transcendence mediated by the idea of a profession ultimately is insufficient to sustain the full transcendent meaning of medicine, it is a gesture toward this transcendence and carries some of its weight.

Professing Medicine

The swearing of an oath is part of what makes medicine "special."[8] It is part of what *constitutes* medicine as a genuine profession.[9] Physicians do not simply receive a degree. They enter a profession. They do so by speaking the words of a public profession. The professing of these words is a performative utterance, like a christening or other naming ceremony.[10] This swearing is a large part of what makes a professional *professional*. To swear the oath *is* to become the professional.

Many occupations have profession-like characteristics. Few are truly professions in the sense that the traditional three medieval professions—medicine, law, and the ordained ministry—are professions. Abraham Flexner, the great reformer of American medical education, counted the following as characteristics of a profession:

- The profession's activities are essentially intellectual in character (i.e., not manual labor) and are practiced (largely) by individuals for individuals.
- Professions are learned—that is, they are possessed of a specialized body of knowledge that is continually being expanded through research.
- A profession has a practical and socially accepted end for its activities.
- The techniques of a profession are taught through specialized and disciplined training.
- Membership in the profession constitutes membership in a special kind of moral community (Flexner used the term "brotherhood").

- Professions tend toward self-organization and self-regulation.
- Professions expect altruistic motivation from their members.[11]

Members of the three traditional medieval professions do all these things in one form or another. They all swear oaths to do so. Moreover, each of these characteristics of a profession corresponds to one of the moral characteristics of an oath that I describe above. Oaths are commitments to service. The swearing of an oath conditions and contextualizes the altruism and the practical social aim of a profession. Oaths are commitments to honesty. The swearing of an oath conditions and contextualizes the pursuit of specialized knowledge and its practical professional application. Oaths are commitments to accountability. The swearing of an oath conditions and contextualizes the self-regulation of a profession. Persons who swear oaths become different persons. Professionals enter a special moral community through their oaths.

Thus, medicine would seem to be a profession par excellence. The moral foundation of this profession begins because someone who is sick and vulnerable has no choice but to ask other human beings for help and is forced to trust in the person who is providing that help.[12] If that other person is a professional healer who has sworn an oath to work for the good of the sick person, he or she is automatically presumed to be worthy of receiving the trust of the patient. The question is whether anyone can take physicians' oaths seriously enough to trust that this presumption is true.

Physicians' Oaths: Current State of Affairs

From a purely empirical point of view, physicians' oaths do not seem to be taken very seriously today. Few physicians remember what they swore.[13] Graduates take their oaths about as seriously as they take the academic regalia of the graduation. The oath is treated as a vestigial ceremonialism.

It is no longer clear that patients take physicians' oaths seriously either. Their trust in doctors is eroding.[14] Many state legal codes refer to physicians' oaths, deferring to the self-regulating function of the profession even if they do not take it as the state's obligation to define the content of these oaths. Yet state medical boards, by and large, take action against physicians only for the most egregious violations of their oaths. By and large, they do not take physicians' oaths very seriously either.

What Is the Moral Work Involved in Taking an Oath Seriously?

Physicians might be more appreciative of their oaths if they could be more reflective about the spiritual nature of what they do on a daily basis. Physicians have the privilege of entering deeply into people's lives—into the mysteries of life, illness, death, hope, fear, love, grief, and joy. Physicians touch people in intimate places where no one else is allowed to touch them. They learn about patients' darkest secrets and most private joys. Every encounter with every patient can be a transformative experience, if one is attentive to the awesome mysteries that surround each patient encounter. One must allow oneself to be so transformed, however.

Physicians offer patients what they have professed. They put it on the line when they don their white coats. What they do on a daily basis truly is amazing. A physician is *never* simply treating high blood pressure or diabetes. A physician treats Mrs. Jones or Mr. Smith—each an individual human person who suffers uniquely the burdens imposed by diabetes or high blood pressure. Treating each individual is an intellectual endeavor. Treatments evolve rapidly through research. A physician must be a lifelong learner of new knowledge. The specialized professional end toward which the physician strives, however, is always the same in every clinical encounter—a right and good healing act for *this* patient in these circumstances.[15] One is taught how to do this through the words and examples of one's teachers. One then becomes privileged to be part of a moral community committed to the care of patients. This community is singularly noteworthy for professing a dedication to altruistic service by means of an oath. Medicine is a true profession. Physicians who understand this foundation might begin to take their oaths more seriously.

Oaths and the Ethics of Virtue

The central moral concern of an oath is that individuals who take the oath swear to be certain kinds of persons. They do not merely recite a laundry list of do's and don'ts, and they do not guarantee a certain type of outcome. Oaths are more about the character of the agents who swear them than their actions.

This characteristic is not true simply of physicians' oaths; it is a characteristic of all oaths. Persons who enlist in the military, for instance, swear an oath, and that oath also does not list specifics. It does not say, "I will never intentionally harm innocent noncombatants" or "I will never flee from battle unless given the order to retreat." It says, "I will support and defend the Constitution of the United States against all enemies, foreign and domestic; I will bear true faith and allegiance to the same." This oath describes a total orientation of the person toward a moral ideal.

Consequently, the ethics of an oath ought to be the ethics of virtue—virtues such as altruism, fidelity, compassion, and competence. Hence I am not bothered so much that some of the specific moral precepts of the traditional Hippocratic Oath are not mentioned in the modified Hippocratic Oaths sworn at many medical schools. There are a great variety of oaths now in common use: the traditional Hippocratic Oath, modified versions of the Hippocratic Oath, the Declaration of Geneva, the International Code of Medical Ethics, the Prayer of Maimonides, and the Oath of Dr. Louis Lasagna. These oaths differ in content.[16] Most have dropped the traditional Hippocratic commitment to confidentiality and the prohibitions on abortion, euthanasia, and sexual relationships with patients. Personally, I subscribe to all of these traditional moral precepts and hope that they would be accepted once again with renewed vigor by the medical profession worldwide. That is an argument for another time and venue, however. What matters most—the point of departure—is to establish the importance that oath-swearing holds for the meaning and integrity of medicine as a profession. This is the sense in which oaths have spiritual importance, mediating important aspects of the transcendent meaning of medicine. What seems to be essential in any medical oath is the commitment to dedicate oneself to the professional characteristics of medicine that transcend the individual practitioner—to lifelong learning, to teaching, to the pursuit of truth, and to membership in a moral community dedicated to healing in a spirit of altruistic service.

Specific moral rules provide only a moral floor below which one should not venture. The ethics of an oath, as an ethics of virtue, points to a transcendent ideal (toward moral perfection) and demands a sincere effort to strive toward this ideal.

In professional ethics, rules are not enough. A physician who never breaks a patient's confidentiality, never commits euthanasia, and never sleeps with a patient might still be a miserable doctor who really didn't care much about patients, greedily saw patients as sources of income, and used them exclusively as such without ever recognizing them as genuine persons. Most people want more from their physicians than that. Most people want their physicians to ask more of themselves.

Neither are outcomes enough. A physician who always has perfectly good outcomes (for instance, a surgeon who never loses a patient and successfully cures all gall bladder disease and appendicitis) might still be a miserable doctor if the physician were indifferent toward the plight of patients, never listened to their concerns, and used them merely as a pretext for the display of the physician's intellectual and technical prowess. Most people want more from their physicians than that. Most people want their physicians to ask more of themselves.

A genuine oath calls any person who swears it to an ethics of virtue. It calls each to be a different sort of person. Unless they are hypocrites, the words medical students speak at graduation ought to make them different sorts of persons.

Attacks on Oath-Taking and Professionalism

Broadly speaking, persons who tend to be skeptical about the meaning of physicians' oaths tend to be those who are skeptical about spirituality in medicine. This link, I suspect, is based on a fundamental uneasiness about the notion of transcendence, although it is rarely made explicit. Instead, the skeptics have raised arguments against taking physicians' oaths seriously that are practical and philosophical. To be fair, I must consider some of these arguments on their own merits and explain why I think they are misguided.

Against Professionalism

The concept of professionalism in medicine, as Flexner understood it, is now under fierce attack. Sociologists dismiss professionalism as elitism.[17] Some critics suggest that holding physicians to a higher moral standard than other sorts of persons amounts to hubris. Berlant has even charged that "professionalism" amounts to a carefully disguised front masking a concerted effort at maintaining monopolistic financial control over the health care industry.[18] Popular cartoons ridicule the Oath of Hippocrates as the Oath of Hypocrisy.

Such criticisms misunderstand the meaning of an oath. An oath does not automatically make a person morally better. Nor does failure to live up to the standards of an oath mean that the only purpose of the oath is to deceive the public before whom it is sworn. An oath simply sets a new moral standard—generally higher than that expected of the general public.

The first way an oath sets a higher moral standard is by raising the floor of moral expectation. Many of the role-specific expectations of professionals would be considered heroic in other occupations. This characterization in no way implies that Mary is a morally better person than John simply because she is a doctor and he is a professor of comparative literature. Taking the Oath of Hippocrates neither implies that Mary will reach heaven before John nor that she is purposefully *feigning* sincerity in what she swears. However, saying that Mary is a doctor means that we have certain role-specific expectations of her that we would consider heroic for John. For example, if Mary is a surgeon, we expect that Mary will get out of bed at 3 AM to remove John's gangrenous appendix. If Mary does not do so, she is not a good doctor. On the other hand, if John's student has a burning question the night before the exam at 3 AM, we do not expect that John will get out of his bed and rush over to the student's house to explain it all carefully. If John were to do so, John would be considered a heroically devoted teacher. Conversely, if John said, "Wait until morning," we would not consider John a bad teacher.

The second sense in which the moral standard for professionals can be said to be higher is the expectation that professionals will exert significant personal effort to reach virtuous ideals as part of their role-specific morality. To examine why this is so, consider an example of two people's failure to exert effort to be virtuous in their work. Suppose that both Mary and Fred are technically excellent at what they do. Mary's patients always survive surgery, the problem is always fixed, and they never have any complications. Her neighbor, Fred, is an animal exterminator. If anyone ever has raccoons living in the attic, Fred is the man to get rid of them quickly, cleanly, and efficiently. Suppose, however, that Mary is always brusque and egotistical, never expresses concern about her patients, and always overcharges them. We would consider her deficient *as a physician*. If Fred is always brusque and egotistical, never expresses concern for his customers, and always overcharges them, we would certainly consider him deficient *as a person*, but we would not consider him deficient as an exterminator. This difference is subtle, but real. The role of the professional calls for a standard of virtue that affects the individual's standing *qua* professional in a way that other occupations do not require.

Finally, there is a sense in which the moral expectations of professionals can even go beyond their role-specific duties and virtues. The Oath of Hippocrates refers to this concept obliquely, stating, "I will live a good and holy life." Consider the following example. Mary has another neighbor named Joe who is a real estate dealer. Mary and Joe would both be said to have behaved wrongly if they had engaged in nefarious behavior outside their professional roles. Suppose both had engaged in insider trading on pork futures, amassing huge fortunes. I suspect that the degree of outrage from the average person regarding the same action would be greater toward Mary than toward Joe. Why?

Because Mary would be regarded as having betrayed professional moral expectations. She has already been well remunerated by a society that wanted to reward its professionals well. Most members of society would consider Mary's behavior a mark of ingratitude toward them. Furthermore, she would be considered to have invested money that came from their flesh, not just from their bank accounts. The outrage would be greater because she had profiteered with money gained from the misfortunes of others. The moral expectations imposed on physicians have a wider penumbra than the expectations imposed on other occupations.

Again, I am not asserting that the professional moral standards that physicians swear to uphold magically make them morally superior human beings. I am suggesting that only the most fuzzy-minded sort of egalitarianism would call it elitist to suggest that there are such things as role-specific moral standards. Many occupations have role-specific moral standards that are higher than those of other occupations. Persons who provide essential services—police and fire department workers, for instance—are not allowed to go on strike. This prohibition does not mean that police officers and fire fighters are morally better than other workers who are allowed to strike—only that their roles are different.

Furthermore, the fact that some ne'er-do-wells hide behind the mask of role-specific moral standards does not imply that the moral standards behind which they hide are evil. Politicians, for instance, regularly transform roles of public service into opportunities to accumulate power and wealth. This phenomenon does not mean that calling politicians back to roles of service is immoral. Similarly, one might justifiably charge that physicians historically have used their professional privileges to their own advantage rather than that of their patients or the public. Yet this indictment does not imply that it is immoral to call physicians to greater accountability—for living up to the high standards to which they have sworn.

Setting role-specific moral standards for professionals is important for at least three reasons. First, taking an oath to uphold such standards *does* establish these role-specific duties and expectations of virtuous behavior. Second, setting such standards may help to attract the right persons to the professions. Third, if one takes these expectations seriously, one is justified in trying to inculcate such virtues in persons who train for the profession.

Against Hippocratic Ethics

The ancient Hippocratic Oath certainly is controversial in our morally pluralistic society. The original oath prohibits abortion, euthanasia, and sexual relationships with patients. Some ethicists consider the oath "unilateral," "gratuitous," "paternalistic," and "irrelevant" to today's medico-moral world.[19] In a world of moral pluralism, critics of the oath say, there can be no such thing as a universal professional ethic.[20] Therefore, they argue, there can be no real oath.

Questioning the moral content of the physician's oath and making arguments that this content ought to be changed is legitimate. This acknowledgment does not imply, however, that the entire idea of oath-taking is morally misplaced. That the laws of a nation might be considered immoral is not an argument that lawmaking ought to be abandoned in favor of anarchy. Of course, whether physicians should swear an oath is open to debate. My point is that disagreement with the moral content of a particular oath does not constitute an argument against oath-taking of some sort. Nor does moral pluralism preclude the possibility that there might be some core moral content of an oath to which all members of society could agree.

Moral Irrelevance of Oaths

Although almost all U.S. medical schools require graduates to take some sort of oath, few schools these days actually have them swear the original Oath of Hippocrates.[21] Critics point to a trend toward schools requiring swearing of oaths that have progressively less substantive content. There are few particular moral precepts in these oaths, except perhaps confidentiality—which actually is the most difficult to practice. There is little content to these oaths. Why, then, bother swearing one?

Other critics charge that even if one were to grant the oath substantial moral content, physicians wouldn't necessarily change their behaviors.[22] Taking oaths didn't stop Nazi physicians from committing all sorts of horrendous crimes against humanity. If oaths could not deter the Nazis and generally seem unenforceable, why bother to swear them?

Furthermore, skeptics ask, where are the data showing that oaths make any difference in health care outcomes? Outcomes dominate the thinking of our implicitly utilitarian society. Thus, the only important question one can ask, according to some observers, is, "What difference do oaths make?"[23] Only the actions of doctors and the results of their actions seem to count. Whatever someone says, or even swears, simply doesn't matter. What matters is how doctors behave. So, some critics seem to say, in effect, "Dispense with the oath. Spare me all the pious nonsense."[24]

Persons who make these arguments do have some valid points. Yet these criticisms do not seem to amount to an argument to abandon the practice of oath-taking altogether. First, granting that the content of oaths has become watered down, there are alternatives to abandonment of the practice of oath-taking. One could reexpand and strengthen the moral content of the oath physicians swear or try to distill the most essential moral content and include that content in a universal medical oath. Second, the Nazi experience cuts both ways. One might argue that the fact that oaths have not been taken seriously is precisely what leads to such atrocities. Perhaps if Nazi physicians had taken their oaths seriously—or if German society had taken the oaths of its physicians seriously—some or all of these medical atrocities might have been prevented.

Third, arguments against oath-taking that are based on an implicitly utilitarian mindset can be rebutted. There are at least two ways to do this without arguing against the ethical propriety of utilitarianism per se. First, many morally reflective persons are not utilitarians. Utilitarians cannot impose utilitarian ethical analysis on everyone. Many nonutilitarians believe that keeping one's word is a good thing, independent of the consequences. They believe in the moral meaning of states of character or virtue. They hold that honoring one's oath is a moral imperative independent of the outcomes. Their views cannot be ignored. Second, one could construct a utilitarian argument that the net social good would be served by having a rule requiring physicians to swear oaths. In the long run, taking these oaths seriously and enforcing them will result in a world in which physicians do the right thing consistently and patients can trust that such behavior will be forthcoming from their physicians. This dynamic would appear to increase net social happiness. Hence, even a utilitarian ought to agree that oath-taking by physicians is morally justifiable, provided that the practice is taken seriously.

Finally, one should be aware that medicine may be the last bastion of positivism (the philosophical view that whatever cannot be empirically verified by sense data can be dismissed as utter nonsense). Many criticisms of oath-taking have a distinctly positivistic flavor. For some of these critics, apparently, the notion that anything at all actually happens simply because someone swears an oath is to be discounted as utter nonsense. For multiple reasons, however, this position is very strange. First, language must have meaning. Otherwise, arguments that oaths are meaningless themselves must be discounted as meaningless. Second, if language does have meaning, perhaps the first principle of morality is that one should be true to one's word. Isn't honesty, the keeping of one's word, morally valuable, even on utilitarian grounds? Third, oaths do appear to form important and new relationships between people and their words, in the special way I have noted.

No one is arguing that taking an oath automatically changes someone's character. If language and human relationships are real, however, an oath does change something about interpersonal relationships and the moral standards to which one is held. To accept oath-taking as meaningful requires belief in the moral dynamics of language and interpersonal relationships. Anyone who doubts that the complex relationship between persons and their words is morally meaningful doubts that morality is meaningful.

Essential Moral Content of a Physician's Oath

If oaths are meaningful, what sort of oath should physicians swear? Given the fact that the specific moral content of oaths has been gradually watered down over the years, some observers have suggested that a restoration effort is in order.[25] Others argue that critiques of the content of the Oath of Hippocrates and the intense moral pluralism of our society imply that physicians could never agree about what oath they should swear, and oath-taking therefore ought to be abandoned.[26]

It will be very difficult, if not impossible, either to restore the original Hippocratic Oath or to craft a revised oath stipulating a very specific set of controversial moral precepts that will be morally acceptable to all physicians. For example, the original oath prohibited abortion. Even schools that now claim to use the original oath simply delete this prohibition. The original oath also prohibited assisted suicide. How could physicians swear this oath in Oregon, where assisted suicide is legal? Restoration of an oath with this sort of moral content simply would be impossible today.

Therefore, one faces three types of alternatives. First, one might concede to those who recommend abandoning oath-taking altogether. One might base this concession on the conclusion that fashioning any sort of universally acceptable oath with any sort of real moral content is impossible. I think this kind of concession is too drastic, however. One should not give up on the idea of oath-taking altogether simply because there are diverse views about the particulars of medical morality. Given all that I have discussed about spirituality, transcendence, professionalism, and virtue, clearly it is too important that physicians should commit themselves to a certain core moral identity.

A second alternative would be to allow various groups of physicians to establish new medico-moral communities, swear various types of oaths or none at all, and hope that one such community might spring up, flourish, and produce an oath that will last through the next millennium or two. That is what happened in ancient Greece. One peculiar sect of physicians on the island of Cos, inspired by a man named Hippocrates, distinguished itself from among the many alternative kinds of

Greek medicine practiced in the fifth century BCE and began to swear an oath. Eventually, they set the scientific and moral standards for medicine.

I am not yet prepared to abandon the hope that there is enough common moral ground remaining among physicians to craft a single oath for all of them. I believe that one might be able to formulate an oath with robust moral content that would maintain continuity with the Hippocratic tradition and bring that powerful and important approach forward into the twenty-first century. Although the Hippocratic tradition of oath-taking might need to evolve, perhaps it does not need to be completely abandoned.

Therefore, one might consider a third alternative. One might try to fashion an oath that has genuine moral content and is in continuity with the Hippocratic tradition but avoids specifying the most controversial particular moral precepts. For instance, one could still ask physicians to swear to put patient service above personal gain but avoid the thorny issue of forswearing abortion. The moral particulars of an oath might not be as important as the moral act of profession itself—professing an oath to transcend one's particularity, to uphold all the moral criteria that distinguish the profession, and in that process to become a professional. Hence, at least a few important general moral precepts could be incorporated into such an oath with universal approbation.

A universal medical ethic with specific precepts is not impossible. On the contrary, such an ethic *is* possible. The oath that physicians swear need not contain the entirety of medical ethics, however. What matters most is the general moral content of the oath. The reason I am not as concerned about the particular moral precepts of the oath as about the fact of *taking* an oath is that, as I argue above, the ethics associated with oath-taking is the ethics of virtue, not the ethics of duty or of outcomes. In any physicians' oath worth its salt, physicians should swear to commit themselves to the service of their patients—putting patients' interests first. They should swear to pursue their profession with intellectual honesty and moral integrity. They should do so in a formal, public manner and declare themselves accountable for what they have sworn. The precise do's and don'ts are simply not as important. An oath can refer to a code of ethics; properly speaking, however, an oath ought not *be* a code of ethics. One can argue about the details of such a code later. First, grant that physicians ought to be swearing an oath at all.

One commonly used oath commits persons who swear it to work for "the good of the sick . . . to the utmost of [their] powers." These graduates solemnly pledge to exercise the art "solely for the cure of [their] patients and the prevention of disease." That is, they swear to put the health of their patients first, committing themselves formally to altruistic service and integrity. This attitude is a crucial part of what distinguishes a physician from a shoemaker, investor, teacher, craftsman, or scientist. I do not mean to suggest that these occupations are immoral or that shoemakers, for example, can't be altruistic. I simply mean that medicine is different. It requires a higher moral standard. The oath is the formal mechanism by which this standard is set. It is a performative utterance by graduates, witnessed by their teachers, families, and friends. It invokes a transcendent witness. It instantiates the transcendence of a profession. If it is taken seriously, the oath changes the moral expectations and relationships between medical school graduates and society.

Concrete Implications

Taking physicians' oaths seriously would have multiple concrete implications. These implications would be morally significant. Some practitioners might even consider these implications dangerous to their own self-interest. That is precisely the point.

These concrete implications might include the following:

- Evaluation of character might become a more prominent part of the process of selecting students for medical school. Schools must consider the question, "Does this person appear to have the compassion, integrity, interpersonal skills, and humility necessary to become a good physician?" Fear of bias or lawsuits often limits this approach in practice, but innovative approaches are being suggested.[27] Empowering admissions offices to make decisions according to some such criteria, rather than according to academic record and board scores alone, would be helpful.

- In recent years, a new practice has emerged in which students who begin medical school officially receive their white coats in a rite of initiation known as a "White Coat Ceremony."[28] Although such practices vary considerably, many schools apparently ask matriculating medical students to swear the Oath of Hippocrates as part of this ceremony.[29] If physicians' oaths truly were taken seriously, however, students would not swear the oath at a ceremony that takes place upon matriculation. If the oath were taken seriously, students would have to earn the right to take it and defer swearing the oath until graduation. They would need to prove that they had not only the intellectual skills and knowledge but also the necessary virtue. They certainly could receive their white coats at a White Coat Ceremony. They could be reminded of the nobility of the undertaking they have begun. They could be asked to attest to their willingness to abide by some sort of moral code of conduct for students. They could even be told, as they begin medical school, about the content of the oath they would hope to swear at the conclusion of their years of study. If the oath were truly understood as a performative utterance, however, by which people who merely hold medical degrees became true physicians, they would not actually swear the oath because they would not yet be certified to be physicians.

- Asking that medical schools be transformed into "schools for virtue" would become legitimate. These days, such a proposal probably would be treated with derision, in part because physicians' oaths are not taken seriously. Passing exams is all that tends to count. Efforts are under way, however, to bolster opportunities for medical students to be exposed to physician-teachers who would exemplify and cultivate among students and trainees virtues appropriate to being a physician. Many observers have been distressed at the erosion of idealism in medical students over their course of studies.[30] They bemoan the subtle way in which students learn most about how to behave from the cues they pick up from house officer and faculty behavior. They learn quickly the kinds of behaviors for which they are rewarded by these powerful individuals, who pay little attention to the kinds of things taught in first- or second-year medical student ethics courses.[31] Courses in ethics, now common in medical schools, are necessary but not sufficient. If medical schools were to take the oath seriously, they also would foster student development in virtue. They would make sure that their graduates were capable of the virtues they are to profess at graduation. After all, medical schools are asked to testify that graduates have not only passed their tests but also have developed the moral and interpersonal skills necessary to merit the swearing of this oath. As a related consequence, medical schools should be empowered to expel students for failing to act in accord with the moral standards of the profession, or at least be able to bar graduates from practice for failing to have the sort of character for which the oath calls.

- The profession would take self-regulation more seriously. Current ethical standards established by professional organizations regarding this aspect of professionalism, even on paper, barely amount to more than a promise to report colleagues who have engaged in criminal activities. Even this standard is almost never enforced. State medical boards (rather than professional societies or one's colleagues in a local institution) provide a potential means for upholding professional moral standards, but even this mechanism tends to be used only as an alternative to pressing criminal charges against physicians whose misconduct has been frankly criminal. If the profession and the public were to take physicians' oaths and the professional concept of self-regulation seriously, hospital medical boards, local medical societies, and state medical boards would begin to call physicians to meet the moral standards of the profession. This kind of accountability might worry some physicians. Genuine professionalism demands genuine self-regulation and sincere public accountability, however. If physicians' oaths were taken seriously, this spirit would need to be restored.
- Physicians would voluntarily forfeit the right to strike or perform any work action that would have a negative impact on their patients. I understand the economic and political developments that have led physicians to entertain this idea. One cannot credibly reassert one's professionalism, however, by acting unprofessionally. Anyone who swears to put the good of patients first cannot use patients as a bargaining tool. Physicians, as true professionals, also would voluntarily forfeit the right to organize through collective bargaining mechanisms for anything other than the purposes of improving patient care services.

Why Do You Want to Be a Doctor?

Most college students on the medical school interview trail are asked repeatedly, "Why do you want to be a doctor?" Curiously, once their medical school interviews are behind them, it is extremely unlikely that anyone will ever ask them this question again. They won't be asked why they want to be a doctor when they move from preclinical science courses to the wards in their third year of medical school. They won't be asked when they graduate. They won't be asked while they are on the interview trail again for internships. They won't be asked when they apply for a license. They won't be asked when they apply for a position in a new practice.

"Why do you want to be a doctor?" I suspect most physicians actually remember what they said during their medical school interviews. If they think hard enough, they probably recall that they mumbled some carefully rehearsed words that sounded a lot like the oath they eventually swore at graduation. The words they spoke probably were words about service to humanity; about love for people; about the search for scientific truth; about a desire to combine scientific knowledge with genuine, caring, intimate human interactions; about how they felt compelled to make the most of the gifts and talents with which they had been blessed and to make a return for those gifts.

My challenge to my fellow physicians and to every medical student in these turbulent times is this: Believe in what you said during your interviews and in what you will swear or have already sworn. Make your declaration truly solemn and intentional. Take it seriously. Don't lose the original idealism you brought to medical school. The profession needs your idealism, your fervor, your zeal. Medicine needs your *spirit*. Don't let it be beaten out of you by a system that can be demanding (at times, too demanding). Resist the temptation toward cynicism. Don't let faceless bureaucrats and financiers make you believe that you are incapable of virtue. Don't be like the tired ones among us who long ago abandoned the ideals that brought them to medicine. Remember why you came. Mean what you say. Do not make your oath subservient to power, markets, politics, or polls. Answer instead to whatever you hold most sacred. Let no one dissuade you from persevering in your idealism to the end of your careers. Don't sell your Hippocratic souls to anyone.

Physicians are ordinary persons. They are called to reach beyond the ordinary, however, toward a transcendent ideal. They are called to

a life of virtue in a profession that is dedicated to a common purpose—
the care of sick persons. This enterprise is inherently moral, in large
part because physicians declare it to be so by the oath they swear at
graduation. Physicians and the society they serve should learn to take
physicians' oaths seriously.

Notes

1. The most widely cited translation of the Oath of Hippocrates is that of Ludwig Edelstein, "The Hippocratic Oath: Text, Translation, and Interpretation," in *Ancient Medicine: Selected Papers of Ludwig Edelstein*, ed. Owsei Temkin and C. Lillian Temkin (Baltimore: Johns Hopkins University Press, 1943), 3–63. For an attempt to relate the oath to the contemporary medical scene, see Steven H. Miles, *The Hippocratic Oath and the Ethics of Medicine* (New York: Oxford University Press, 2003).

2. Robert L. Lowes, "Is the Hippocratic Oath Still Relevant?" *Medical Economics* 72 (June 12, 1995): 197–206; Linda Beecham and Jane Smith, "Report on the Annual Representatives Meeting of the British Medical Associations in Harrogate, July 3, 1995," *British Medical Journal* 311 (1995): 196.

3. Daniel P. Sulmasy, "What Is an Oath and Why Should a Physician Swear One?" *Theoretical Medicine and Bioethics* 20 (1999): 329–46.

4. Immanuel Kant, *Grounding for the Metaphysics of Morals*, Ak. 402–3, trans. James W. Ellington (Indianapolis: Hackett, 1981), 14–15.

5. W. D. Ross, *The Right and the Good* (Oxford: Clarendon Press, 1930), 16–47.

6. Sharon L. Holland, "Section II: Societies of Apostolic Life (Canon 731)," in *The Code of Canon Law: A Text and Commentary*, ed. James A. Corriden, Thomas J. Green, and Donald E. Heintschal (New York: Paulist Press, 1985), 534–35; J. F. Hite, "Title II: Religious Institutes (Canon 607)," in *The Code of Canon Law: A Text and Commentary*, ed. James A. Corriden, Thomas J. Green, and Donald E. Heintschal (New York: Paulist Press, 1985), 407–8.

7. Robert D. Orr, Norman Pang, Edmund D. Pellegrino, and Mark Siegler, "The Use of the Hippocratic Oath: A Review of 20th Century Practice and a Content Analysis of Oaths Administered in Medical Schools in the U.S. and Canada in 1993," *Journal of Clinical Ethics* 8 (1997): 377–88.

8. Daniel P. Sulmasy, "What's So Special about Medicine?" *Theoretical Medicine* 14 (1993): 27–42.

9. Leon R. Kass, "Professing Ethically: On the Place of Ethics in Defining Medicine," *Journal of the American Medical Association* 249 (1983): 1305–10.

10. John L. Austin, "Performative Utterances," in *Philosophical Papers*, 2nd ed., ed. J. O. Urmson and G. J. Warnock (Oxford: Oxford University Press, 1970), 233–52.

11. Abraham Flexner, "Is Social Work a Profession?" *School and Society* 1 (1915): 901–11.

12. Edmund D. Pellegrino and David C. Thomasma, *A Philosophical Basis of Medical Practice* (New York: Oxford University Press, 1981), 192–220.

13. Daniel P. Sulmasy, Eric S. Marx, and Maureen Dwyer, "Knowledge, Confidence, and Attitudes about Medical Ethics: How Do Faculty and Housestaff Compare?" *Academic Medicine* 70 (1995): 1038–40; A. Yakir and Shimon M. Glick, "Medical Students' Attitudes to the Physician's Oath," *Medical Education* 32 (1998): 133–37.

14. A. C. Kao, D. C. Green, A. M. Zaslevsky, J. P. Koplan, and P. D. Cleary, "The Relationship between Method of Physician Payment and Patient Trust," *Journal of the American Medical Association* 280 (1998): 1708–14.

15. Pellegrino and Thomasma, *Philosophical Basis of Medical Practice.*

16. Carol Mason Spicer, "Appendix: Codes, Oaths and Directives Related to Bioethics," in *Encyclopedia of Bioethics*, 2nd ed., ed. Warren T. Reich (New York: Macmillan, 1995), 2599–2842.

17. Eliot Friedson, *Professional Dominance: The Social Structure of Medical Care* (Chicago: Atherton Press, 1970).

18. Jeffrey Lionel Berlant, *Profession and Monopoly: A Study of Medicine in the United States and Great Britain* (Berkeley: University of California Press, 1975).

19. Bernard Lo, *Resolving Ethical Dilemmas: A Guide for Clinicians* (Baltimore: Williams and Wilkins, 1995), 12.

20. Robert M. Veatch and Carol G. Mason, "Hippocratic vs. Judeo-Christian Medical Ethics: Principles in Conflict," *Journal of Religious Ethics* 15 (1987): 86–105.

21. Orr et al., "The Use of the Hippocratic Oath."

22. Friedson, *Professional Dominance.*

23. Irvine Loudon, "The Hippocratic Oath," *British Medical Journal* 309 (1994): 952.

24. Lowes, "Is the Hippocratic Oath Still Relevant?"; Beecham and Smith, "Report on Annual Representatives Meeting."

25. G. Merikas, "Hippocrates: Still Our Contemporary," *Humane Medicine* 8 (1992): 212–18; Brian Hurwitz and Ruth Richardson, "Swearing to Care: The Resurgence of Interest in Medical Oaths," *British Medical Journal* 315 (1997): 1671–74.

26. Lowes, "Is the Hippocratic Oath Still Relevant?"; Beecham and Smith, "Report on Annual Representatives Meeting."

27. Kevin Eva, Harold I. Reiter, Jack Rosenfeld, and Geoffrey R. Norman, "The Relationship between Interviewers' Characteristics and Ratings Assigned during a Multiple Mini-Interview," *Academic Medicine* 79 (2004): 602–9.

28. William T. Branch, "Deconstructing the White Coat," *Annals of Internal Medicine* 129 (1998): 740–41; Bernard Gavzer, "Are the New Doctors Better?" *Parade Magazine* (June 8, 1997), 8–9.

29. Stanley J. Reiser and John C. Ribble, "Oath-Taking at Medical Graduation: The Right Thing at the Wrong Time," *Academic Medicine* 70 (1995): 857–58.

30. Dimitri A. Christakis and Chris Feudtner, "Ethics in a Short White Coat: The Ethical Dilemmas that Medical Students Confront," *Academic Medicine* 68 (1993): 249–54.

31. Edward M. Hundert, Fred Hafferty, and Dimitri A. Christakis, "Characteristics of the Informal Curriculum and Trainees' Ethical Choices," *Academic Medicine* 71 (1996): 624–42.

Part II

The Book of Numbers: Empirical Research on Spirituality and Healing

Recently there has been a dramatic increase in the volume of research about spirituality published in the medical literature. Much of this research looks like other medical research—questionnaires, psychological instruments, recordings of pulse and blood pressure, measurements of immune function, P-values, confidence intervals, and regression analysis. Medical researchers do what they are good at doing, even if the subject is novel.

In part II of this book I reflect on this empirical research effort. Although these research projects represent, in part, early signs of the spiritual rebirth of medicine I have described, little of this research has been systematically evaluated from a theological and spiritual point of view. "Review articles" have summarized the findings of these published research reports. Critics have suggested that all of it is "bunk." My aim is to probe a bit deeper. In chapter 7 I provide an overview, suggesting some important caveats to bear in mind in reviewing empirical studies about spirituality in health care. In chapter 8, I suggest a comprehensive philosophical framework within which to situate empirical research about spirituality in medicine and to summarize and critique some of the available research instruments. In chapter 9 I provide a detailed scientific and theological critique of a small subset of these empirical studies—those assessing the effects of intercessory prayer on clinical outcomes for patients. In chapter 10 I return to themes from Part I and argue that despite my critiques about some of this empirical research, there is a moral imperative for clinicians to address the spiritual needs of patients. Using my analysis of the proper use of empirical research about spirituality I argue that, contrary to much that has been written, data play only a limited role in establishing such an imperative. Some of what these empirical investigators have discovered undoubtedly is true. We need more reflection on what it means, however, as well as why clinicians should care in the first place.

$$\sim\!\!\mathbb{Q} \quad 7$$

What the Data Cannot Mean

One of the major barriers to effective discussion about spirituality, religion, and health care has been improper use of data. Much of this confusion has been fueled by a set of deep, scarcely conscious, background suppositions about the relationship between medical practice and outcomes that has grasped hold of health care today. This set of presuppositions has been reinforced and even amplified by the total quality management and evidence-based medicine movements. In this brief chapter I make some simple but critical cautionary remarks about the pitfalls one ought to avoid in interpreting empirical data about spirituality and health care. I discuss many of these points in more detail in subsequent chapters in this part of the book.

Everyone in health care seems to be enamored of data. Medical schools love data. Funding sources love data. Faculty members love data. Students love data. The government loves data. Insurers love data. Many patients also love data. (Patients who really love data often come to the doctor's office with reams of printouts from their exhausting—though far from exhaustive or focused—data-mining expeditions in cyberspace.)

In this setting, it seems natural to turn to data to grab the attention of health care professionals to convince them of the importance of spirituality and religion and the role they can play in health care. Some proponents of the spirituality and medicine movement seem persuaded that the best way to convince their colleagues that spirituality and religion really have something to contribute to medicine is to "show them the data." Perhaps only data will convince funding agencies that they have spent their money wisely in promoting the role of spirituality in health care.

We must be extremely careful, however, about how we interpret and use data about the roles of spirituality and religion in health care. At least the following five caveats seem important:

- Beware the naturalistic fallacy.
- Association is not causation.
- Prayer is harder to control than gravity.
- Infinity wreaks havoc with both numerators and denominators.
- In God's eyes, "bad" outcomes sometimes are good.

The reader deserves to learn more about the concrete concerns each of these phrases is intended to convey.

Beware the Naturalistic Fallacy

The naturalistic fallacy sometimes is known as the is/ought or fact/value distinction. It is a widely accepted rule of ethics. Roughly, it means that brute facts about the world do not entail moral conclusions.[1] One aspect of this fact/value distinction is almost universally accepted: Believing that one can derive moral prescriptions directly from empirical studies—whether they demonstrate patient satisfaction with spiritual services or describe positron emission tomographic images of patients who are meditating—is simply fallacious. A survey that suggests that 99 percent of patients want their physicians to address spirituality or religion with them is not a sufficient moral warrant for doing so. Such a fact might suggest that one ought to have good reasons for not doing so. Such a fact might motivate one to change one's ways of practicing. This sort of fact does not imply a prescriptive statement, however. If 99 percent of cancer patients were to demand treatment with laetrile, this finding would not imply that physicians have an obligation to supply it. I am not asserting that prayer is like laetrile—only that surveys about patient preferences do not imply, of themselves, any obligation to satisfy those preferences. In both cases, the proposed intervention requires further scrutiny. One would need the permission of individual patients to initiate spiritual or religious discussions or interventions. Patient desire is not itself sufficient, however, to create a moral duty.

Association Is Not Causation

Careful investigators have conducted multiple studies in several settings, controlling well for confounding factors, that demonstrate an association between attendance at worship services and longevity.[2] Although I find these studies convincing, one must be very careful in interpreting what this association means. The fact that people who go to church live longer does not imply that if any particular individual goes to church, that person will live longer. It does not even imply that a population of people who start going to church will, on average, live longer than a similar population of people who do not go to church. There may be something about persons who choose to go to churches, mosques, temples, and synagogues that makes them live longer. This conclusion is just as valid as the conclusion that going to churches, mosques, temples, and synagogues somehow makes them live longer. Alternatively, there may be factors about the activity of attending worship services that may help people live longer that might not be particular to this activity—such as the beneficial physiological effects of prayer and meditation; the sense of discipline, meaning, and hope; the effects of social support; and others—that make the difference.[3] Finally, invoking again the naturalistic fallacy, although this fact is very interesting, it is not a moral warrant for a physician's prescription to go to church. Celibate nuns do not get cervical cancer. No one takes this fact as a moral warrant for physicians to tell patients, "Get thee to a nunnery." (I discuss the moral implications of the data in greater detail in chapter 10.)

Prayer and Gravity

Data on the efficacy of intercessory prayer at a distance are flawed empirically and theologically. Prayer is harder to control than gravity. It goes on whether investigators randomly assign patients to be prayed for or not. There are serious questions about how to measure it. Moreover, making God into just another therapeutic intervention in the doctor's black bag surely must seem blasphemous to a believer. In my view, this entire line of research lacks any scientific or theological merit. (I discuss the topic of randomized trials of intercessory prayer in greater detail in chapter 9.)

Quantifying the Infinite

Many well-intentioned people are trying to develop all sorts of scales to measure various aspects of spirituality and religion in health care. As I discuss in chapter 8, some of these measurement tools have a useful, if limited, place in health care. One can readily measure preferences and behaviors such as attendance at worship services. One can measure religiosity, religious behaviors, and styles of religious coping. Knowing that a dying patient's self-assessed quality of life often is dominated by the patient's spiritual state also is important; very sick patients with only days to live may rate the quality of their lives quite highly.[4]

Things get tricky, however, when one moves into other domains. Reconciliation, transcendent meaning, and hope are substantially harder to quantify. As I discuss in more detail in chapter 8, if the spiritual is truly transcendent, how can one reduce it to a number? Once one unleashes the infinite into one's equations, calculations cease. Some investigators probably are pursuing such quantification because they really do not believe in the transcendent and want to reduce spirituality to a series of measurable psychological states. Other investigators claim to believe in the transcendent yet have become so steeped in the quantifiable world of medicine that in their zealous attempt to justify their faith to their skeptical colleagues through empirical research they betray the fact that their own faith in numbers has become deeper than their faith in God. Their hearts might be with God, but they have already sold their minds to the secularists with whom they would do battle. Such a split between mind and heart is a very unhealthy spiritual state, although I confess that I have no idea how one would try to measure it.

Spirituality and Outcomes

The pragmatist and utilitarian habits of American culture have affected American medicine deeply. Everything today must be justified by its outcome. Few observers appreciate the infinite regress to which such thinking ultimately leads. If everything has value only in terms of its consequences, nothing will ever have value in itself. When our American obsession with outcomes is applied to spirituality in health care, the madness of the obsession seems more evident.

The demand for outcomes data regarding spirituality in health care is a danger not only for physicians and nurses but also for chaplains and pastoral care departments in hospitals. Once pastoral care services succumb to the need to prove, for example, that they can decrease length of stay, improve patient satisfaction, or affect biomedical outcomes, all will be lost.

Sometimes the spiritual will require a dark night of the soul. If a chaplain's visit helps a patient who is dying see that he has been a miserable wretch and the patient comes to feel deep regret over what he has done in his life, the patient's level of spiritual distress might be greater than when he was wallowing in his usual state of smug complacency. Would this outcome be good or bad? If the average patient has a shorter life expectancy after a spiritual intervention, is that fact necessarily bad? In one case it might mean that the patient had accepted death, in another that the patient had sunk into deep despair.

Demanding this sort of evidence to justify spiritual or religious interventions is nonsense. Picasso's masterpiece "Guernica" ought to make us sick when we confront our potential for massive inhumanity.

Yet just as no one ought to demand that art either improve people's moods or increase their productivity on the job, all the more so religions ought to resist the demand to have their importance reduced to such banality.

Data about religion and spirituality do have a place in medical research, teaching, and practice. That place is limited, however, and health care professionals who would use data to convince their skeptical colleagues or students of the importance of spirituality and religion in health care must be very careful to avoid these pitfalls.

Notes

1. Although I support a version of ethical naturalism, I also believe that the naturalistic fallacy has been overextended as a principle in ethics and that knowing something about human nature is critical to the enterprise of doing ethics. This knowing, however, can be accomplished only through logic, ontology, and philosophical anthropology, not through data. See Henry B. Veatch, *For an Ontology of Morals* (Evanston, Ill.: Northwestern University Press, 1971), 99–124.

2. Robert A. Hummer, Richard G. Rogers, Charles B. Nam, and Christopher G. Ellison, "Religious Involvement and U.S. Adult Mortality," *Demography* 36 (1999): 273–85; Harold G. Koenig, Judith C. Hayes, David B. Larson, Linda K. George, Harvey J. Cohen, Michael E. McCullough, Keith G. Meador, and Dan G. Blazer, "Does Religious Attendance Prolong Survival? A Six-Year Follow-Up Study of 3,968 Older Adults," *Journal of Gerontology,* series A, 54, no. 7 (1999): M370–76; J. LeBron McBride, Gary Arthur, Robin Brooks, and Lloyd Pilkington. "The Relationship between a Patient's Spirituality and Health Experiences," *Family Medicine* 30 (1998): 122–26; Douglas Oman and Dwayne Reed, "Religion and Mortality among the Community-Dwelling Elderly," *American Journal of Public Health* 88 (1998): 1469–75; William J. Strawbridge, Richard D. Cohen, Sara J. Shema, and George A. Kaplan, "Frequent Attendance at Religious Services and Mortality over 28 Years," *American Journal of Public Health* 87 (1997): 957–61.

3. Dale A. Matthews and Connie Clark. *The Faith Factor* (New York: Viking Press, 1998), 40–52.

4. S. Robin Cohen, Balfour M. Mount, Eduardo Bruera, Marcel Provost, Jocelyn Rowe, and Kevin Tong, "Validity of the McGill Quality of Life Questionnaire in the Palliative Care Setting: A Multi-Centre Canadian Study Demonstrating the Importance of the Existential Domain," *Palliative Medicine* 11 (1997): 3–20.

8

A Biopsychosocial-Spiritual Model of Health Care

As I argue in part I of this book, finitude is a defining feature of human beings. In fact, we might even say that the fundamental task of medicine, nursing, and the other health care professions is to minister to suffering occasioned by the necessary physical finitude of human persons, in their living and in their dying.[1]

Today's health professions seem to have become superb at addressing the physical finitude of the human body. Previously lethal diseases have become curable or have been transformed into chronic illnesses. In many cases medical progress has been remarkable. What previously was extraordinary now is routine. For example, soon after his inauguration as the vice president of the United States in January 2001, Dick Cheney had a fourth myocardial infarction; an automatic, implantable, cardioverter defibrillator was inserted into his chest, and the public seemed only to yawn.[2] Cheney is still alive five years later.

Despite all this technological progress, contemporary medicine still stands justly accused of having failed to address itself to the needs of whole human persons and preferring to limit its attention to the finitude of human bodies.[3] My purpose in this chapter is to advance a more comprehensive model to guide empirical research about the role of spirituality in clinical care.

Many people are very interested in research about spirituality and health care. The field has developed helter-skelter, however, and lacks a theoretical structure. Building on the themes in Part I of this book, I advance such a theory, assuming patients to be human beings in their wholeness—as persons oriented to the infinite, grappling with their finitude. One may call this conception a biopsychosocial-spiritual model of care. Within this model, one may delineate a circumscribed but very important role for empirical research about spirituality in health care. As part of this effort, I provide a scientific critique of questionnaires and psychological instruments that researchers have used to conduct empirical studies of the role of spirituality in health care and suggest a research agenda for this field.

More Inclusive Models

In the 1970s George Engel laid out a vast alternative vision for health care when he described his biopsychosocial model.[4] This model, not yet fully realized, placed the patient squarely within a nexus that included affective and other psychological states of that patient as a human person, as well as significant interpersonal relationships that surround that person. At about the same time, Kerr White was introducing an ecological model of patient care that included attention to the patient's environment as well—a public health model of primary care.[5] Neither of these models had anything to say about either spirituality or death. Furthermore, although both models asserted certain truths about patients as human persons, neither provided any genuine grounding for these theories in what might be called a philosophical anthropology. That is, neither attempted to articulate a metaphysical grounding for their notions of patients as persons, although both seemed to depend on such a notion.

Both of these models have struggled to find a place in mainstream medicine, in large measure because the successes of medicine have come about by embracing exactly the opposite model. Rather than considering the patient as a subject situated within a nexus of relationships, medical science often has considered the patient as an object amenable to detached, disinterested investigation. Through scientific reduction of the person to a specimen composed of systems, organs, cells, organelles, biochemical reactions, and a genome, medicine has made remarkable discoveries that have led to countless therapeutic advances.

No one disputes that these advances have been positive. Yet the experience of patients and practitioners alike at the dawn of the twenty-first century is that the reductivist, scientific model is inadequate to the real needs of patients who are persons. Cracking the genetic code has not led us to understand who human beings are, what suffering and death mean, what may stand as a source of hope, what we mean by death with dignity, or what we may learn from seriously ill persons. Although all human persons *have* genomes, human persons are not reducible to their genomes. To paraphrase Marcel, a person is not a problem to be solved but a mystery in which to dwell.[6] Holding together in the medical act both the reductivist scientific truths that are so beneficial and the larger truths about the patient as a human person is the enormous challenge health care faces today.

Spirituality and the Medical Model

A few physicians recently have written about the need for a model that goes even further—a biopsychosocial-spiritual model of health care.[7] On closer reading, however, one finds that these authors have merely asserted the need for this expanded model, without doing much more than assigning a name to it. They have not founded it on a philosophical anthropology, and they have not shown how this new model can be reconciled with the contemporary reductivist, scientific conception of the patient or how it can be integrated into a more general metaphysics of life and death.

An entire "movement" has now arisen promoting integration of spirituality into medicine. This movement is split into two camps, neither of which appears adequate to the task of providing a robust theory to guide research. One of these camps discounts the reductivist, scientific model of medicine as "rational," "Western," "biased," "narrow," "chauvinistic," and perhaps even toxic and seeks either to replace it or, at least, to complement it as a parallel universe of medical practice and discourse.[8] The other camp thoroughly accepts the reductivist, scientific model, and although it might extend the boundaries of the scientific model of the patient to include the psychological and the epidemiological, it almost appears to advocate reduction of the spiritual to the scientific.[9] These scientific models of spirituality in health care have produced a startling array of measurement techniques, with very interesting results, but they also have engendered significant confusion over what is being measured, why it is being pursued, and what it means.

I therefore propose some elements of a philosophical anthropology that I hope is adequate to the task of providing a foundation or groundwork for a biopsychosocial-spiritual model of health care. This model brings together multiple themes from Part I of this book, using them as building blocks for this foundation. Only then do I suggest an empirical research agenda regarding spirituality and health care—one that acknowledges and is informed by its limitations.

Spirituality and Religion

As I note in chapter 2, spirituality is a broader term than religion.[10] Spirituality refers to an individual's or group's relationship with the transcendent, however that concept may be construed. Spirituality is about the search for transcendent meaning. Most people express their spirituality in religious practice. Others express their spirituality exclusively in their relationships with nature, music, the arts, or a set of philosophical beliefs or relationships with friends and family. Religion, on the other hand, is a set of beliefs, practices, and language that characterizes a community that is searching for transcendent meaning in a particular way, generally on the basis of belief in a deity. Thus, although not everyone has a religion, everyone who searches for ultimate or transcendent meaning can be said to have a spirituality.

The Human Person: A Being in Relationship

The cornerstone of the philosophical anthropology I propose is the concept of the human person as a being in relationship. Because each person is in relationship with the transcendent—even if by way of rejecting the very possibility of transcendence—human persons are intrinsically spiritual.

From a philosophical point of view, one can argue that being *is* relationship. To know a thing (literally, any "thing") is to grasp the complex set of relationships that define it, whether that thing is a bacterium or a human being.[11] This argument is all the more true of living things. Hans Jonas has put it this way: "Being thus suspended in possibility is through and through a fact of polarity, and life always exhibits it in these basic respects: the polarity of being and not-being, of self and world, of form and matter, of freedom and necessity. These, as is easily seen, are forms of relation: life is essentially relationship; and relation as such implies 'transcendence,' a going-beyond-itself on the part of that which entertains the relation."[12]

Disease can be described as a disruption of right relationships. It is not "looking at a bad body inside an otherwise healthy body." *Clostridium dificile* colitis is not a bad body one sees under a microscope. The disease is not identical with the bacterium. The disease is a disturbance in the relationships that ought to prevail within the colon of a human being. A disease is always a disruption in right relationship.

Contemporary scientific healing retains the same formal structure that informed prescientific cultures: Healing is still about the restoration of right relationships. This, healing, however, ought not be limited to restoration of the homeostatic relationships of the patient as an individual organism. Illness disturbs more than relationships *inside* the human organism. It also disrupts families and workplaces. It shatters preexisting patterns of coping. It raises questions about one's relationship with the transcendent.

Thus, one can say (figure 8.1) that illness disturbs relationships both inside and outside the body of the human person. Inside the body, the disturbances are twofold: They affect relationships between and

Figure 8.1. Illness and the Manifold of Relationships of the Patient as a
Human Person

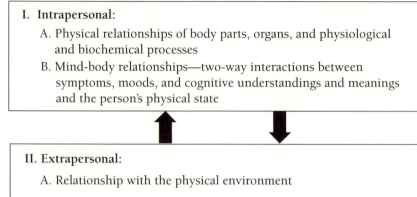

I. Intrapersonal:
    A. Physical relationships of body parts, organs, and physiological
       and biochemical processes
    B. Mind-body relationships—two-way interactions between
       symptoms, moods, and cognitive understandings and meanings
       and the person's physical state

II. Extrapersonal:
    A. Relationship with the physical environment
    B. Relationship with the interpersonal environment—family, friends,
       communities, political order
    C. Relationship with the transcendent

among the various body parts and biochemical processes and the relationship between the mind and the body. Outside the body, these disturbances also are twofold: They affect the relationship between the
individual patient and his or her environment—including the ecological, physical, familial, social, and political nexus of relationships surrounding the patient—and the relationship between the patient and the
transcendent.

Healing the Whole Person

In this model, healing can be defined even more precisely than by vague
references to "making whole" that I make in chapter 2. Healing, in its
most basic sense, means restoration of right relationships. Genuinely
holistic health care is a system of health care that attends to all of the
disturbed relationships of the ill person as a whole, restoring those that
can be restored, even if the person is not thereby completely restored

to perfect wholeness. A holistic approach to healing means that correction of physiological disturbances and restoration of the *milieu interior* is only the beginning of the task. Holistic healing requires attention to psychological, social, and spiritual disturbances as well. As Teilhard de Chardin insists, besides the *milieu interior* there also is a *milieu divin*.[13]

Furthermore, even when cure is no longer possible—when the *milieu interior* no longer can be restored—healing is still possible, and the healing professions still have a role. No matter what the patient's spiritual history, serious illness raises for the patient questions about the value and meaning of his or her life, suffering, and death. These questions are obvious—they are about meaning, value, and relationship.[14]

Therefore, appropriate care of seriously ill persons requires attention to restoration of all the intrapersonal and extrapersonal relationships that can still be addressed, even when the patient is dying. Considering the relationship between mind and body in its broadest sense, symptomatic treatment restores the human person by relieving him or her of the experiences of pain, nausea, dyspnea, fatigue, anxiety, and depression. Considering the relationship between the human person and the environment, genuine healing means, for example, facilitation of reconciliation with family and friends within the biopsychosocial-spiritual model. When the seriously ill individual experiences love, is understood as valuable even when he or she no longer is economically productive, and accepts the role of teacher by providing valuable lessons to those who provide care, that person experiences healing. Finally, when questions about existence, meaning, value, and relationship arise in the context of health care, they are starkly circumscribed by the finitude that disease, injury, and death make manifest. Healing, in a complete sense, must involve the overriding question of whether the answers to these perennial questions transcend that finitude.

If the human person is essentially a being in relationship, then even the person who has chosen to believe that there is no such thing as transcendence has made a choice in relationship to that question, which is put before each of us. Each person must live and die according to the answer each gives to the question of whether life or death has a meaning that transcends both life and death. In this model, facilitation of a patient's grappling with such questions is an act of healing.

The Biopsychosocial-Spiritual Model of Care

According to this model, everyone has a spiritual history. For many persons, this spiritual history unfolds within the context of an explicit religious tradition. Regardless of how this spiritual history has unfolded, however, it helps shape each patient as a whole person; when life-threatening illness strikes, it strikes each person in his or her totality.[15] This totality includes not only the biological, psychological, and social aspects of the person but the spiritual aspects of the whole person as well.[16] This biopsychosocial-spiritual model is not a "dualism" in which a "soul" accidentally inhabits a body. In this model, the biological, psychological, social, and spiritual are distinct dimensions of the person, and no individual aspect can be disaggregated from the whole. Each aspect can be affected differently by a person's history and illness, and each aspect can interact and affect other aspects of the person.

Do Patients Want Clinicians to Address Their Spiritual Concerns?

All this theorizing might be moot if patients were uninterested in medical attention to their spiritual concerns. Initial research suggests, however, that between 41 percent and 94 percent of patients want their physicians to address these issues.[17] In one survey, even half of the nonreligious patients thought that physicians should inquire politely about patients' spiritual needs.[18] These findings are particularly true if patients are at the end of life or are more religious to begin with.[19] These results also are corroborated by surveys regarding patients' desire for nursing attention to their spiritual concerns.[20] Nonetheless, if patients reply that they do not have spiritual or religious concerns or do not wish them to be addressed in the context of the clinical relationship, respect for the patient's freedom and dignity suggests that the clinician must always respect the patient's refusal.[21]

Physicians generally are reluctant to address patients' spiritual concerns in practice.[22] In one study, oncologists rated the importance of spiritual distress low compared with seventeen other clinical concerns they felt they were responsible for addressing.[23] In addition, studies have shown that health care professionals fail to address the spiritual needs of patients with "do not resuscitate" (DNR) orders. Physicians make referrals to chaplains or otherwise address the spiritual needs of patients with DNR orders less than 1 percent of the time.[24]

Can One Measure a Patient's Relationship with the Transcendent?

One can only measure what can be measured. This statement appears to be trivial, but investigators often neglect its truth.

God is a mystery. This recognition does not mean that one cannot know God. It does mean that the way in which one knows God transcends the spatiotemporal limits on which empirical measurement depends. In addition, the Abrahamic religious traditions, if not all religious traditions, teach that the way God speaks to the human heart leaves ultimate judgments to God, not to other human beings. Thus, the very idea of measuring spiritual awareness, spiritual need, spiritual distress, death transcendence, or religious coping poses a variety of theological questions.[25]

Nonetheless, patients and researchers readily identify particular attitudes, aspects of human distress, ways of coping, and particular behaviors as religious or spiritual. These attitudes, beliefs, feelings, and behaviors are amenable to measurement. As long as investigators are careful to understand the extremely limited view these measurements give of the spiritual life, and as long as clinicians are properly reticent about using these measurements in caring for individual patients, these tools have their place. Above all, they can help institutions and pro-

grams determine, in a general way, whether they are responding appropriately to the needs of their patients.

What Domains Might Be Measured?

In measuring the measurable aspects of spirituality and religion, we can
usefully distinguish which aspect is being assessed. I have suggested the
following four distinct categories:

- Religiosity (e.g., strength of belief, prayer and worship practices, intrinsic versus extrinsic)
- Spiritual/religious coping and support (e.g., response to stress in terms
  of spiritual language, attitudes, practices, and sources of spiritual
  support)
- Spiritual well-being (e.g., spiritual state or level of spiritual distress as a
  dimension of quality of life)
- Spiritual needs (e.g., conversation, prayer, ritual; over what spiritual
  issues?).[26]

Although there can be a tendency to lump all of these categories together, they all serve different purposes.

Religiosity

Religiosity has been the most extensively studied of the four domains.
Religiosity is itself complex and can be said to consist of many dimensions, such as denominational preference, religious beliefs, values,
commitment, organizational religiosity, private religious practices, and
daily spiritual experiences. The report of the Fetzer Institute/National
Institute on Aging Working Group on measures of religiosity provides
a unique and important resource, tabulating and evaluating multiple
instruments—many of which have been evaluated extensively for validity, reliability, and other psychometric properties.[27] This group also has
proposed a single composite, multidimensional instrument to measure
religiosity.

Among these many dimensions of religiosity, a patient's religious denomination has had the least predictive value in health care research. The most consistently predictive items have measured specific behaviors, such as church attendance, prayer, or reading of sacred texts. Other dimensions that research has shown correlate with health and health care include attitudes such as self-described strength of religious belief.[28]

Research has shown that religiosity has significant predictive value in health care research. Multiple studies have linked religiosity to improved long-term health outcomes, even when the researchers have controlled their statistical models for smoking, alcohol and drug use, and other potential confounders.[29] There is little information, however, about linkages between religiosity and end-of-life care.

One promising new and unique measure is Daily Spiritual Experience.[30] This instrument, which has undergone extensive psychometric study, asks subjects to quantify—from "never" to "many times a day"—daily experiences such as closeness to God, gratitude to God, sense of religious peace, and dependence on God for assistance. Daily spiritual experience is related to decreased alcohol use, improved quality of life, and positive psychosocial state.

Researchers also have developed instruments to classify persons according to the important distinction between intrinsic and extrinsic religiosity. Intrinsic religiosity refers to "living" a religion—practicing and believing for the sake of the religion. Extrinsic religiosity refers to "using" a religion—practicing and espousing beliefs for the sake of something else, such as getting a certain job or being seen as a certain type of person.[31] Intrinsic religiosity has been linked to lower death anxiety.[32] Many other useful studies might be undertaken to examine how religiosity affects aspects of health care. Investigators should be cautious, however, in asking about the link between religiosity and health care outcomes. For example, intensely religious patients may have become too debilitated to attend religious services. Although prior religiosity might predict the seriously ill patient's present state, few data would suggest fresh ideas about how knowing this information might help practitioners in caring for patients.

Spiritual/Religious Coping and Support

Perhaps more important in the care of seriously ill persons is to understand their current manner of religious coping, rather than their past religious beliefs, practices, and attitudes. Religious coping refers to how one's spiritual or religious beliefs, attitudes, and practices affect one's reaction to stressful life events. Few instruments measure this coping, although the RCOPE and INSPIRIT both have track records.[33] The former is more purely a measure of religious coping, the latter a measure of more general spiritual coping. Assessing what sort of inner resources the patient has for dealing with the stress of terminal illness seems very relevant to the care of seriously ill persons. Importantly, these instruments measure both positive (e.g., acceptance or peace) and negative (e.g., excessive guilt or anger) religious coping mechanisms. A measure of religiosity might or might not be associated with a person's religious coping style.

Religious *coping* measures a person's internal resources and reactions. Religious *support* measures the resources and reactions of the religious community that can be mustered on behalf of a patient. Religious support can be considered a subset of social support.[34] There are no validated instruments to measure this construct, however.

Spiritual Well-Being

The World Health Organization (WHO) has declared that spirituality is an important dimension of quality of life.[35] Quality of life consists of multiple facets. How one is faring spiritually affects one's physical, psychological, and interpersonal states, and vice versa. All contribute to one's overall quality of life. Thus, trying to measure spiritual well-being—or its opposite, spiritual distress—is particularly useful. These characteristics can be measured as discrete end points in themselves or as subscales contributing to one's quality of life. All of these spiritual well-being measures are descriptions of the patient's spiritual state of affairs, which can function as an outcome measure or as an independent variable potentially associated with other outcomes. For example, a patient's spiritual history, present religious coping style, and present biopsychosocial state, as well as any spiritual intervention, would combine to affect the person's present state of spiritual well-being, which in turn would contribute to the person's overall quality of life.

To date, the most rigorously studied of the available instruments appears to be the FACIT-SP.[36] Related instruments include the Spiritual Well-Being Scale and the Meaning in Life Scale.[37] The McGill Quality of Life Questionnaire has a very useful spiritual well-being subscale and has been developed specifically for patients at the end of life.[38] The Death Transcendence scale looks specifically at spiritual issues related to dying.[39]

Some of these instruments have been criticized as confounding spiritual well-being with psychological well-being, but the critics appear to have confounded for themselves measurement of spiritual well-being and measurement of religiosity.[40] All of these instruments have their advantages and disadvantages. Mytko and Knight, as well as Puchalski, have prepared excellent reviews of these instruments.[41] Although the individual instruments vary quite a bit, one very important message is that the phenomena they measure account for a substantial part of the variance in patients' overall quality-of-life ratings that cannot be reduced to other measures of psychosocial well-being and coping.[42]

Spiritual Needs

Clinically, measures of the religious/spiritual *needs* of patients at the end of life may be more important than measures of religiosity or religious coping, and these measures avoid all potential controversy about the meaning of a patient's spiritual state as an outcome measure. Qualitative studies have suggested that patients have many such spiritual needs.[43] Unfortunately, few instruments are available. Moadal and coworkers have developed such an instrument, but it has yet to undergo psychometric testing.[44] Pastoral care professionals also have taken some steps toward constructing measures of spiritual need that might be of help to physicians.[45]

The Complex Interaction of These Domains

For clinical and research purposes, it is important to see how various measurement domains regarding spirituality interact and which might serve as dependent or independent variables. As figure 8.2 depicts, this new model suggests that the patient comes to the clinical encounter with a spiritual history, a manner of spiritual/religious coping, a state of spiritual well-being, and concrete spiritual needs. Some of these states serve as independent variables, predicting how the patient will fare spiritually in the face of illness. In addition, according to this model, this spiritual state may be modulated by the biopsychosocial state of the person, and the spiritual state may modulate the biopsycho-social state. The composite state—how the patient feels physically, how the patient is faring psychologically and interpersonally, as well as how the patient is progressing spiritually—constitutes the substrate of the construct we call quality of life. Although quality of life might be mea-surable, we also must understand that "quality of life is not just a vari-able. It is where we live."[46] In the care of persons at the end of life, the biopsychosocial-spiritual state of the patient is the ground upon which that patient lives until death and the ground from which that person posits himself or herself into whatever there is after death—whether absolute annihilation or beatific bliss.

Figure 8.2. The Biopsychosocial-Spiritual Model of the Care of Patients

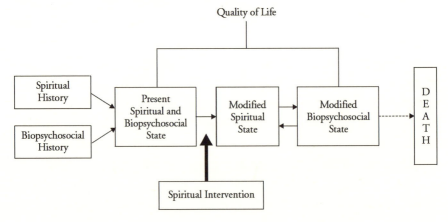

For research purposes, either quality of life or the spiritual component of quality of life (spiritual well-being) might be the outcome variable of interest in an intervention study. As figure 8.2 shows, for example, an experimental spiritual intervention (e.g., a new, standardized spiritual assessment of each patient by clergy) might modify the spiritual well-being of the person. In studying this outcome, however, one also might need to control for spiritual history, religious coping, and physical and psychological states. Alternatively, one might be interested in studying the effects of a spiritual intervention on the biopsychosocial state of the patient. Figure 8.2 provides a framework for examining these complex interactions.

A Research Agenda

Although more has been accomplished in this field than most investigators realize, much work remains to be done. I believe that the following areas are important topics for further research in the nexus of spirituality and health care.

Measuring Value and Meaning (Dignity and Hope)

There appear to be no well-developed measures of patients' own sense of either dignity or hope. Nonetheless, measures of spiritual well-being (as well as measures of quality of life that include a spiritual dimension) almost always include items referring to these concepts. Investigators ought to have no preconceptions about dignity or hope to which the patient must conform. Even among patients with the same religion, the particularity of individual spiritualities would preclude this sort of preconceptualizing. Some preliminary work, using semantic differential techniques to develop an empirical model for hope, has recently been undertaken.[47] Another good instrument is the Herth Hope Index.[48] Both of these approaches are commendable because they focus on a hope that is much broader than mere biomedical prognosis. Harvey Chochinov has begun similar work regarding an empirical construct for dignity.[49] Because these features are key to the spiritual growth of seriously ill patients, more work should be done to refine these constructs and to create new instruments that might concentrate on these dimensions.

Whose Role?

Who should facilitate the patient's spiritual healing? The fact that patients have said in surveys that they want doctors to be involved does not mean that the proper roles have been assigned. What are the proper roles of family and friends? What is the proper role of clergy and pastoral care? What is the proper role of the nurse or physician? What are the views of believing and nonbelieving patients about these roles? How should all these parties interact, if at all? We need to know more about what all of these prospective spiritual agents believe, what they might be capable of accomplishing, and what will be most effective for patients.

Interactions between the Four Domains of Spirituality and Other Measures

I have set forth a classification scheme of measures of patient spirituality, yet almost nothing is known about the interactions among these domains. For example, does prior patient religiosity (presumably intrinsic) predict better spiritual well-being at the end of life? Does better spiritual coping predict less spiritual distress? Does better spiritual well-being predict more or less spiritual need? Which of the many dimensions of religiosity are most important? Furthermore, although large population-based outcome studies have associated religiosity with mortality, the field appears to be wide open for research that examines the relationship between these four domains of spirituality and phenomena such as ethical decision making, symptom severity, site of death, and more.

Effectiveness of Spiritual Interventions

As one might imagine, there are almost no data regarding the "effectiveness" of spiritual or religious interventions in the care of patients. In one British survey of a random sample of relatives of deceased patients, 63 percent of these survivors stated that their loved one's religious faith was of help to the patient at the time of death, regardless of belief in an afterlife.[50] This finding, however, does not answer the question of whether spiritual or religious interventions by health care professionals might make a difference. One randomized controlled trial integrates attention to spiritual issues in the psychotherapeutic care of patients with cancer, but the results have not been published as of this writing.[51]

Several studies have investigated whether prayer at a distance or other nonphysical spiritual, complementary, or alternative interventions can affect health care outcomes.[52] These studies have been highly controversial, and the efficacy of these interventions has not been firmly established or disproved.[53] I discuss these studies in much greater detail in chapter 9.

Spiritual Significance of Patient–Professional Relationships

Research should pay attention to the importance of the relationship between the health professional and the patient as a possible context for the patient to work out and express spiritual concerns and struggles. For example, Rachel Remen tells the story of a patient who does not want any more chemotherapy but enjoys the support of his oncologist so much that he keeps asking for more chemotherapy because he fears losing that relationship if he "stopped the chemo."[54]

Again, this field of research appears to be wide open. Are better relationships associated with better spiritual well-being scores or spiritual coping? Does the relationship with the health care professional affect spiritual needs? These and related questions would be interesting inquiries for research.

Tools for Taking Spiritual Histories

Numerous mnemonic devices have been developed for clinicians who are inexperienced at taking a spiritual history. The purpose of these devices is to help clinicians remember what questions to ask patients regarding spirituality, and how to ask them—similar to the CAGE questions for screening for alcoholism.[55] One acronym is HOPE; the H stands for sources of hope, O is for the role of organized religion, P is for personal spirituality and practices, and E is for effects on care and decision making.[56] In the acronym FICA, F stands for faith and beliefs, I is for the importance of spirituality in your life, C is for spiritual community of support, and A is for how the patient wishes these issues to be addressed.[57] In a third acronym, SPIRIT, S stands for spiritual belief system, P is for personal spirituality, I is for integration with a spiritual community, R is for ritualized practices and restrictions, I is for implications for medical care, and T is for terminal events planning.[58] My personal practice is to allow much of this discussion to unfold by using a simple open-ended question: "What role does spirituality or religion play in your life?"

These history-taking tools are strikingly similar, even though they have been developed independently. None, however, has undergone any serious psychometric testing. The questions are relevant to understanding the lives and spiritual needs of patients, and one might argue that such psychometric testing is no more necessary than validating how to ask questions about past medical history, occupation, sexual practices, and hobbies. Nevertheless, development of valid and predictive instruments for clinicians would be a useful field of study.

For research purposes, George has proposed a measure of spiritual history in the sense of spiritual development and life history—a construct that is distinct from, although closely related to, the clinical sense of the word *history*.[59] This instrument is based on previously developed questionnaires, none of which has been extensively validated, so there is ample opportunity for work in this area as well.

Role of the Professional's Own Spirituality

Clinicians should pay attention to the spiritual lessons that seriously ill persons can teach them.[60] Because the word "doctor" means "teacher," this attitude is a bit of a role reversal. Yet a sick person needs to understand his or her value. Seriously ill patients have a role in teaching us, even when they have become "unproductive."

I have suggested previously that clinicians need to pay attention to their own spiritual histories and be conscious of how this history affects the care they give their patients.[61] This consciousness seems especially important in caring for patients at the end of life.[62] There are no studies, however, to support the idea that practitioners' histories affect the care they provide. An interesting research approach would be to administer instruments measuring the four domains to physicians and other health care professionals and explore how their scores affect the care they deliver.

Spirituality after Death

Grieving families and friends have spiritual needs, spiritual/religious coping mechanisms, and measurable degrees of religiosity. The ways in which these factors affect bereavement would be a fascinating topic for study. Another interesting area of study would be to begin to understand more about the role of spiritual well-being in the bereavement processes and its role within the overall quality of life of persons who survive their loved ones. Finally, research into how the spirituality of the deceased patient affects the bereavement of those who survive him or her also would be interesting. Little work has been done in this area.

Humanities Research

Empirical studies, including qualitative empirical studies, offer only a very limited view of spirituality. The fields of philosophy of religion, theology, comparative religions, history, literature, and the arts have far more to say about the core of spirituality than do descriptive studies. One excellent way to begin to bridge the gap between twenty-first-century medicine and the world of spirituality and religion might be to advance a research agenda that is open to funding investigation of spirituality and health care that uses the techniques of these disciplines in the humanities.

Conclusions

A human person is a being in relationship—biologically, psychologically, socially, and transcendently. The patient is a human person. Illness disrupts all of the dimensions of relationship that constitute the patient as a human person. Therefore, only a biopsychosocial-spiritual model can provide a foundation for treating patients holistically. Transcendence itself, by definition, cannot be measured. One can measure patients' religiosity, spiritual/religious coping, spiritual well-being, and spiritual needs, however. A research agenda in this area would include the following:

- Improving measurements of spiritual states
- Better defining who is best able to address these issues with patients
- Studying the interactions between the measurable dimensions of spirituality and more traditional health measures
- Designing and measuring the effectiveness of spiritual interventions
- Assessing the spiritual significance of patient–professional relationships
- Refining and testing tools for taking spiritual histories
- Assessing the impact of the health professional's own spirituality on end-of-life care
- Developing measurement tools for assessing the religious coping, spiritual well-being, and spiritual needs of persons who mourn deceased loved ones
- Encouraging scholarship in the humanities about these issues.

The biopsychosocial-spiritual model I propose in this chapter appears to be rich enough to accommodate this ambitious and exciting research agenda.

Notes

1. Daniel P. Sulmasy, "Finitude, Freedom, and Suffering," in *Pain Seeking Understanding: Suffering, Medicine, and Faith,* ed. Mark J. Hanson and Margaret Mohrman (Cleveland: Pilgrim Press, 1999), 83–102.

2. Edward Walsh and Shankar Vedantam, "Cheney Receives Coronary Implant; Defibrillator to Regulate Heartbeat," *Washington Post* (July 1, 2001), A1.

3. Paul Ramsey, *The Patient as Person* (New Haven, Conn.: Yale University Press, 1970).

4. George L. Engel, "The Need for a New Medical Model: A Challenge for Biomedicine," *Science* 196, no. 4286 (1977):129–36.

5. Kerr L. White, Franklin T. Williams, and Bernard G. Greenberg, "The Ecology of Medical Care," *Bulletin of the New York Academy of Medicine* 73 (1996): 187–212.

6. Gabriel Marcel, *Being and Having*, trans. K. Farrer (Glasgow, Scotland: The University Press, 1949), 117.

7. Dana E. King, *Faith, Spirituality and Medicine: Toward the Making of a Healing Practitioner* (Binghamton, N.Y.: Haworth Pastoral Press, 2000); D. D. McKee and J. N. Chappel, "Spirituality and Medical Practice," *Journal of Family Practice* 35 (1992): 201, 205–8.

8. See, for example, Deepak Chopra, *Perfect Health: The Complete Mind-Body Guide* (New York: Three Rivers Press, 2001); Caroline M. Myss, *Anatomy of the Spirit: The Seven Stages of Power and Healing* (New York: Random House, 1997); Andrew Weil, *Spontaneous Healing: How to Discover and Embrace Your Body's Natural Ability to Maintain and Heal Itself* (New York: Knopf, 1995).

9. See, for example, Dale A. Matthews and Connie Clark, *The Faith Factor* (New York: Viking Press, 1998); H. Benson, M. S. Malhotra, R. F. Goldman, G. D. Jacobs, and P. J. Hopkins, "Three Case Reports of Metabolic and Electroencephalographic Changes during Advanced Buddhist Meditation Techniques," *Behavioral Medicine* 16 (1990): 90–95.

10. Alan B. Astrow, Christina M. Puchalski, and Daniel P. Sulmasy, "Religion, Spirituality, and Health Care: Social, Ethical, and Practical Considerations," *American Journal of Medicine* 110 (2001): 283–87.

11. Bernard J. F. Lonergan, *Insight: A Study of Human Understanding* (San Francisco: Harper and Row, 1958), 245–67.

12. Hans Jonas, *The Phenomenon of Life* (Evanston, Ill.: Northwestern University Press, 2001), 4–5.

13. Pierre Teilhard de Chardin, *The Divine Milieu* (New York: Harper, 1960).

14. Daniel P. Sulmasy, "Is Medicine a Spiritual Practice?" *Academic Medicine* 74 (1999): 1002–5; idem, "Healing the Dying: Spiritual Issues in the Care of the Dying Patient," in *The Health Professional as Friend and Healer*, ed. Judith Kissel and David C. Thomasma (Washington, D.C.: Georgetown University Press, 2000), 188–97; idem, "At Wit's End: Dignity, Forgiveness, and the Care of the Dying," *Journal of General Internal Medicine* 16 (2001): 335–38.

15. Ramsey, *The Patient as Person*.

16. George Engel, "How Much Longer Must Medicine's Science Be Bound by a Seventeenth Century World View?" *Psychotherapy and Psychosomatics* 57, no. 1–2 (1992): 3–16; King, *Faith, Spirituality and Medicine*; King, "Spirituality and Medical Practice."

17. Timothy P. Daaleman and Donald E. Nease, "Patient Attitudes Regarding Physician Inquiry into Spiritual and Religious Issues," *Journal of Family Practice* 39

(1994): 564–68; John W. Ehman, Barbara B. Ott, Thomas H. Short, Ralph C. Ci-ampa, and John Hansen-Flaschen, "Do Patients Want Physicians to Inquire about Their Spiritual or Religious Beliefs If They Become Gravely Ill?" *Archives of Internal Medicine* 159 (1999): 1803–6; Dana E. King and Bruce Bushwick, "Beliefs and Atti-tudes of Hospitalized Patients about Faith Healing and Prayer," *Journal of Family Practice* 39 (1994): 349–52; Alyson Moadel, Carole Morgan, Anne Fatone, Jennifer Grennan, Jean Carter, Gia Laruffa, Anne Skummy, and Janice Dutcher, "Seeking Meaning and Hope: Self-Reported Spiritual and Existential Needs among an Ethni-cally Diverse Cancer Patient Population," *Psycho-Oncology* 8 (1999): 378–85; Charles D. MacLean, Nancy Phifer, Linda Schultz, Deborah Bynum, Mark Franco, Andria Klioze, Michael Monroe, Joanne Garrett, and Sam Cykert, "Patient Prefer-ence for Physician Discussion and Practice of Spirituality," *Journal of General Inter-nal Medicine* 18 (2003): 38–43.

18. Ehman et al., "Do Patients Want Physicians to Inquire about Their Spiritual or Religious Beliefs If They Become Gravely Ill?"

19. Ibid.; Moadel et al., "Seeking Meaning and Hope"; MacLean et al., "Patient Preference for Physician Discussion and Practice of Spirituality"; Daaleman and Nease, "Patient Attitudes Regarding Physician Inquiry into Spiritual and Religious Issues."

20. Pamela Reed, "Preferences for Spiritually Related Nursing Interventions among Terminally Ill and Non-Terminally Ill Hospitalized Adults and Well Adults," *Applied Nursing Research* 4 (1991): 122–28.

21. Daniel P. Sulmasy, "Addressing the Religious and Spiritual Needs of Dying Patients," *Western Journal of Medicine* 175 (2001): 251–54.

22. Mark R. Ellis, Daniel C. Vinson, and Bernard Ewigman, "Addressing Spiri-tual Concerns of Patients: Family Physicians' Attitudes and Practices," *Journal of Family Practice* 48 (1999): 105–9.

23. Jean L. Kristeller, Collette S. Zumbrun, and Robert F. Schilling, "'I Would If I Could': How Oncologists and Oncology Nurses Address Spiritual Distress in Can-cer Patients," *Psycho-Oncology* 8 (1999): 451–58.

24. Daniel P. Sulmasy, Gail Geller, David M. Levine, and Ruth Faden, "The Quality of Mercy: Caring for Patients with Do Not Resuscitate Orders," *Journal of the American Medical Association* 267 (1992): 682–86; Daniel P. Sulmasy and Eric S. Marx, "A Computerized System for Entering Orders to Limit Treatment: Imple-mentation and Evaluation," *Journal of Clinical Ethics* 8 (1997): 258–63; Daniel P. Sulmasy, Eric S. Marx, and Maureen Dwyer, "Do the Ward Notes Reflect the Qual-ity of End-of-Life Care?" *Journal of Medical Ethics* 22 (1996): 344–48.

25. Sulmasy, "Healing the Dying."

26. Ibid.

27. Fetzer Institute/National Institute on Aging Working Group, *Multidimen-sional Measurement of Religiousness/Spirituality for Use in Health Research* (Kalama-zoo, Mich.: Fetzer Institute, 1999).

28. Ibid.

29. Robert A. Hummer, Richard G. Rogers, Charles B. Nam, and Christopher G. Ellison, "Religious Involvement and U.S. Adult Mortality," *Demography* 36 (1999): 273–85; Harold G. Koenig, Judith C. Hayes, David B. Larson, Linda K. George, Harvey J. Cohen, Michael E. McCullough, Keith G. Meader, and Dan G. Blazer, "Does Religious Attendance Prolong Survival? A Six-Year Follow-Up Study of 3,968 Older Adults," *Journal of Gerontology*, series A, 54, no. 7 (1999): M370–76; J. LeBron McBride, Gary Arthur, Robin Brooks, and Lloyd Pilkington, "The Relationship between a Patient's Spirituality and Health Experiences," *Family Medicine* 30 (1998): 122–26; Douglas Oman and Dwayne Reed, "Religion and Mortality among the Community-Dwelling Elderly," *American Journal of Public Health* 88 (1998): 1469–75; William J. Strawbridge, Richard D. Cohen, Sara J. Shema, and George A. Kaplan, "Frequent Attendance at Religious Services and Mortality over 28 Years," *American Journal of Public Health* 87 (1997): 957–61.

30. Lynn G. Underwood and Jean A. Teresi, "The Daily Spiritual Experience Scale: Development, Theoretical Description, Reliability, Exploratory Factor Analysis, and Preliminary Construct Validity Using Health-Related Data," *Annals of Behavioral Medicine* 24 (2002): 22–33.

31. Gordon W. Allport and J. Michael Ross, "Personal Religious Orientation and Prejudice," *Journal of Personality and Social Psychology* 5 (1967): 432–43; Richard L. Gorsuch and Susan E. McPherson, "Intrinsic/Extrinsic Measurement: I/E Revisited and Single-Item Scales," *Journal for the Scientific Study of Religion* 28 (1989): 348–54; Dean R. Hoge, "A Validated Intrinsic Religious Motivation Scale," *Journal for the Scientific Study of Religion* 11 (1972): 369–76.

32. James A. Thorson and F. C. Powell, "Meanings of Death and Intrinsic Religiosity," *Journal of Clinical Psychology* 46 (1990): 379–91.

33. Kenneth I. Pargament, Harold G. Koenig, and Lisa M. Perez, "The Many Methods of Religious Coping: Development and Initial Validation of the RCOPE," *Journal of Clinical Psychology* 56 (2000): 519–43; Larry VandeCreek, Susan Ayres, and Meredith Bassham, "Using INSPIRIT to Conduct Spiritual Assessments," *Journal of Pastoral Care* 49, no. 1 (1995): 83–89.

34. Neal Krause, "Religious Support," in Fetzer Institute/National Institute on Aging Working Group, *Multidimensional Measurement of Religiousness/Spirituality for Use in Health Research*, 57–63.

35. WHOQOL Group, "The WHO Quality of Life Assessment (WHOQOL) Position Paper from the World Health Organization," *Social Science and Medicine* 41 (1995): 1403–9.

36. Marianne J. Brady, Amy H. Peterman, George Fitchett, May Mo, and David Cella, "A Case for Including Spirituality in Quality of Life Measurement in Oncology," *Psycho-Oncology* 8 (1999): 417–28; S. P. Cotton, E. G. Levine, C. M. Fitzpatrick, C. H. Dold, and E. Targ, "Exploring the Relationships among Spiritual Well-Being, Quality of Life, and Psychological Adjustment in Women with Breast Cancer," *Psycho-Oncology* 8 (1999): 429–38.

37. Raymond F. Paloutzian and Craig W. Ellison, "Loneliness, Spiritual Well-Being and Quality of Life," in *Loneliness: A Sourcebook of Current Theory, Research*

and Therapy, ed. Letitia A. Peplau and Daniel Perlman (New York: Wiley, 1982), 224–47; Stephanie C. Warner and J. Ivan Williams, "The Meaning in Life Scale: Determining the Reliability and Validity of a Measure," *Journal of Chronic Diseases* 40 (1987): 503–12.

38. S. Robin Cohen, Balfour M. Mount, Eduardo Bruera, Marcel Provost, Jocelyn Rowe, and Kevin Tong, "Validity of the McGill Quality of Life Questionnaire in the Palliative Care Setting: A Multi-Centre Canadian Study Demonstrating the Importance of the Existential Domain," *Palliative Medicine* 11 (1997): 3–20; S. Robin Cohen, Balfour M. Mount, Michael G. Strobel, and France Bui, "The McGill Quality of Life Questionnaire: A Measure of Quality of Life Appropriate for People with Advanced Disease: A Preliminary Study of Validity and Acceptability," *Palliative Medicine* 9 (1995): 207–19.

39. Larry VandeCreek and Christina Nye, "Testing the Death Transcendence Scale," *Journal for the Scientific Study of Religion* 32 (1993): 279–83.

40. Allen C. Sherman, Thomas G. Plante, Stephanie Simonton, Dawn C. Adams, Casey Harbison, and S. Kay Burris, "A Multidimensional Measure of Religious Involvement for Cancer Patients: The Duke Religious Index," *Supportive Care in Cancer* 8 (2000): 102–9.

41. Johanna J. Mytko and Sara J. Knight, "Body, Mind and Spirit: Towards the Integration of Religiosity and Spirituality in Cancer Quality of Life Research," *Psycho-Oncology* 8 (1999): 439–50; Christina M. Puchalski, "Spirituality," in *Toolkit of Instruments to Measure End-of-Life Care,* ed. Joan Teno (1999); available at www.chcr.brown.edu/pcoc/Spirit.htm (last accessed June 6, 2005).

42. Cohen et al., "Validity of the McGill Quality of Life Questionnaire."

43. Carla P. Hermann, "Spiritual Needs of Dying Patients: A Qualitative Study," *Oncology Nursing Forum* 28 (2001): 67–72.

44. Moadal et al., "Seeking Meaning and Hope."

45. Milton W. Hay, "Principles in Building Spiritual Assessment Tools," *American Journal of Hospice Care* 6 (1989): 25–31.

46. Eric Cassel, comment during medical Grand Rounds, Mayo Clinic, Rochester, Minn., February 14, 2001.

47. Cheryl L. Nekolaichuk, Ronna F. Jevne, and Thomas O. Maguire, "Structuring the Meaning of Hope in Health and Illness," *Social Science and Medicine* 48 (1999): 591–605; Cheryl L. Nekolaichuk and Eduardo Bruera, "Assessing Hope at the End of Life: Validation of an Experience of Hope Scale in Advanced Cancer Patients," *Palliative and Supportive Care* 2 (2004): 243–53.

48. K. Herth, "Abbreviated Instrument to Measure Hope: Development and Psychometric Evaluation," *Journal of Advanced Nursing* 17 (1992): 1251–59; Astrid K. Wahl, Tone Rustoen, Anners Lerdal, Berit R. Harnestad, Øisten Knudsen, and Torbjørn Moum, "The Norwegian Version of the Herth Hope Index (HHI-N): A Psychometric Study," *Palliative and Supportive Care* 2 (2004): 255–63.

49. Harvey Chochinov, "Dignity-Conserving Care: A New Model for Palliative Care," *Journal of the American Medical Association* 287 (2002): 2253–60.

50. Ann Cartwright, "Is Religion a Help around the Time of Death?" *Public Health* 105 (1991): 79–87.

51. Kenneth Pargament and Brenda Cole, "Re-Creating Your Life: A Spiritual/ Psychotherapeutic Intervention for People Diagnosed with Cancer," *Psycho-Oncology* 8 (1999): 395–407.

52. William S. Harris, William S. Manoha Gowda, Jerry W. Kolb, Christopher P. Strychacz, James L. Vacek, Philip G. Jones, Alan Forker, James H. O'Keefe, and Ben D. McCallister, "A Randomized, Controlled Trial of the Effects of Remote, Intercessory Prayer on Outcomes in Patients Admitted to the Coronary Care Unit," *Archives of Internal Medicine* 159 (1999): 2273–78; Randolph C. Byrd, "Positive Therapeutic Effects of Intercessory Prayer in a Coronary Care Unit Population," *Southern Medical Journal* 81 (1988): 826–29.

53. Cynthia B. Cohen, Sondra E. Wheeler, David A. Scott, Barbara Springer Edwards, and Patricia Lusk, "Prayer as Therapy: A Challenge to Both Religious Belief and Professional Ethics," *Hastings Center Report* 30 (May–June 2000): 40–47; John A. Astin, Elaine Harkness, and Edzard Ernst, "The Efficacy of 'Distant Healing': A Systematic Review of Randomized Trials," *Annals of Internal Medicine* 132 (2000): 903–10.

54. Rachel Naomi Remen, *Kitchen Table Wisdom* (New York: Riverhead Books, 1996).

55. C = Have you ever Cut down or thought about Cutting down on alcohol intake? A = Do you ever become Angry when people ask about your drinking? G = Have you ever felt Guilty about anything you did while drinking? E = Do you ever have an Eye-opener to get you going in the morning? See Dennie Mayfield, Gail McLeod, and Patricia Hall, "The CAGE Questionnaire: Validation of a New Alcoholism Screening Instrument," *American Journal of Psychiatry* 131 (1974): 1121–23.

56. Gowri Anandarajah and Ellen Hight, "Spirituality and Medical Practice: Using the HOPE Questions as a Practical Tool for Spiritual Assessment," *American Family Physician* 63 (2001): 81–89.

57. Astrow et al., "Religion, Spirituality, and Health Care"; Steven G. Post, Christina M. Puchalski, and David B. Larson, "Physicians and Patient Spirituality: Professional Boundaries, Competency, and Ethics," *Annals of Internal Medicine* 132 (2000): 578–83.

58. Todd A. Maugans, "The SPIRITual History," *Archives of Family Medicine* 5 (1996): 11–16.

59. Linda K. George, "Religious/Spiritual History," in Fetzer Institute/National Institute on Aging Working Group, *Multidimensional Measurement of Religiousness/ Spirituality for Use in Health Research*, 65–69.

60. Sulmasy, "Healing the Dying"; Alasdair C. MacIntyre, *Dependent Rational Animals: Why Human Beings Need the Virtues* (Chicago: Open Court, 1999), 136–38; Ira Byock, *Dying Well: The Prospect for Growth at the End of Life* (New York: Riverhead Books, 1997); Michael Kearney, *Mortally Wounded* (New York: Scribner, 1996).

61. Daniel P. Sulmasy, *The Healer's Calling: A Spirituality for Physicians and Other Health Care Professionals* (New York: Paulist Press, 1997).

62. Nancy Chambers and J. Randall Curtis, "The Interface of Technology and Spirituality in the ICU," in *Managing Death in the Intensive Care Unit: The Transition from Cure to Comfort,* ed. J. Randall Curtis and Gordon D. Rubenfeld (New York: Oxford University Press, 2001) 193–206; Sulmasy, "Healing the Dying."

9

Scientific Studies of the Healing Power of Prayer

In chapter 8 I propose a broad philosophical, theological, and scientific model for an empirical research program regarding spirituality and health care. I note that although there has been burgeoning interest among practitioners and patients regarding the subject of spirituality and health care, heretofore the whole field has lacked any coherent, carefully thought out theoretical framework. In chapter 8 I attempt to provide the outlines of such a framework, but I also sharply criticize some potential misuses of empirical research about spirituality in health care.

In my critique, I identify some views about the relationship between spirituality and mainstream Western medicine that seem to rest on inauthentic notions of the nature of spirituality. In this chapter, I address one of these misguided viewpoints in detail—the viewpoint that appears to undergird studies that examine the medical effects of intercessory prayer on behalf of patients.

The recent upsurge of interest in medicine and spirituality has engendered a particular interest, in some quarters, in conducting scientific studies of the efficacy of intercessory prayer. I consider in detail four of the most widely cited studies: the 1988 study by Randolph Byrd, the 1997 study by William Harris and colleagues, the 1998 study by Fred Sicher and colleagues, and the 1999 study by Scott Walker and colleagues.[1] All four of these studies were randomized, controlled, clin-

ical trials in which the researchers randomly chose patients to be
prayed for or not be prayed for by groups of outside volunteers who
did not know the patients. Two studies concerned outcomes in cardiac
intensive care units, a third concerned outpatients with advanced AIDS,
and the fourth took place in an alcohol treatment center. Three reported statistically significant positive effects. The alcohol treatment
study showed no effect.

I have no doubt that the investigators who conducted these studies
are sincere. Some may even be quite devout. The studies seem to have
been carefully carried out and honestly reported. I think there are fundamental flaws in these studies, however—scientifically, morally, and
theologically. I do not believe these flaws can be overcome by doing
better science. I believe these sorts of studies are simply misguided from
the outset.

Scientific Critique

At first glance, these studies all seem scientifically rigorous. The randomized, double-blinded, controlled clinical trial is the "gold standard"
for research used to evaluate medical interventions such as new drugs
or new surgical techniques. The four studies I discuss in this chapter
were all randomized, double-blinded, controlled clinical trials. They
suffer from some very important scientific problems, however. The results of these investigations should not be accepted at face value as tele-
vision news "sound bites" about them have suggested to the public.

Randomization and Blinding

The first scientific issue concerns randomization. In a standard randomized clinical trial of a drug, patients consent to be given one of two
different kinds of pills. By a random process, patients are selected to
receive either a pill that contains the actual drug that is being tested or
one that looks identical to the active drug (and ideally even tastes identical) but contains inert ingredients. The latter is known as a placebo.

"Blinding" means that the patients do not know which of these two pills they will receive. "Double-blinding" means that the persons evaluating their clinical response also do not know which type of pill the patients are receiving. Ideally, the persons who are caring for the patients also should be blinded because doctors and nurses also can communicate subtly to patients, even unconsciously, which among them are receiving the experimental intervention—and thereby affect the results. All of the parties involved in any randomized controlled trial are prone to the biases of therapeutic enthusiasm, delight in novelty, and various forms of the placebo effect. Patients who are aware that they are receiving the experimental intervention might subconsciously feel better. Experimenters who knew which patients were receiving the treatment and which were not might be unconsciously disposed to classify borderline results as favorable if they occurred in the treatment group and unfavorable if they occurred in the placebo group. Rigorous blinding procedures guard against such subtle biases because no one will know who is actually receiving the active drug until the experiment is over. Thus, the experiment is "controlled."

As in all science, whatever one learns from such an experiment is *ceteris paribus* knowledge. One hopes that the random process takes care of balancing out all other factors except the drug (such as the proportion of people with a predisposition to develop a rash when taking the drug) and that the only thing that has been done differently between the two groups is administration of the active drug or the placebo.

The four studies I discuss in this chapter were all randomized and double-blinded. Patients were assigned to be the subjects of a prayer group's intercessions or not, at random. The patients and the clinicians evaluating the effects of prayer were all "blind" to who was being prayed for. These design features were all methodologically sound.

There is one possible wrinkle in this assessment with regard to the study by Sicher et al. Although the researchers collecting the data were blinded, it is unclear whether the clinicians who were treating the patients also were blinded. This issue is important because the treating clinicians, even unconsciously, could have signaled to the patients whether they were receiving the active intervention. The treating doctors and nurses also decided on the outcomes of interest, such as which patients would be hospitalized and when the next visit would occur, and they recorded the clinical information that the blinded evaluators abstracted from the patients' charts. Thus, the information may have been recorded according to a subconscious bias, even if it was later evaluated as data in a blinded fashion.

More important, as other critics also have observed, an experiment about prayer cannot prevent patients assigned to the nonprayer group from praying for themselves or having other persons pray for them.[2] This factor would affect any attempt to conduct a randomized study about the effectiveness of prayer. In other words, none of these experiments truly can be controlled properly. People who are assigned to receive a placebo in a study of a new drug have almost no chance of receiving the experimental drug from another source. No one else besides the experimenters has the drug to give to the patients. By contrast, however, most sick people will be prayed for. Religious people often pray for the health of atheists, and Christians are instructed to pray even for their enemies. People pray for recovery for themselves, their relatives, their friends, and their co-workers all the time. Thus, the "placebo group" in such experiments is unlikely to be a placebo group at all.

One might argue that this factor should "balance out" in the randomization process—that equal numbers will be prayed for by others in both groups. This line of reasoning does not resolve the experimenter's problem, however. If 90 percent of both groups are being prayed for, the experiment necessarily will be a failure. Only 10 percent are actually not being prayed for—and thus constitute the true control group—and one does not have a ready way of sorting these persons out. Two consequences follow. First, the true experiment is "underpowered"—there are not enough subjects to make statistical inferences. Second, if one cannot identify who the true control patients are, any actual statistical effect will be diluted because these true control patients are lost in the crowd. One says that such an experiment has been "contaminated."

One might argue further that even if this kind of contamination occurred, one could still use all the data because there would be more people praying for patients in the experimental group. Therefore, prayer should still be more effective for this group. One would need to be able to quantify, however, how many other people were praying for the patients in both groups in addition to the prayers of the experimental prayer group. Discerning these data would be well-nigh impossible.

Operationalizing Prayer as an Experimental Intervention

Furthermore, even thinking about doing this kind of experiment leads to a complicated theological and scientific conundrum. Is there a "dose-response" curve for prayer? Is prayer more effective if more people are praying? Is there a "ceiling effect," so that after a certain "dose" there is no more efficacy? Is there a toxic dose—as with all other medical interventions—such that too much prayer is actually damaging? These questions create an irresolvable dilemma. Even thinking in terms of dose-response curves and toxicity with excess prayer would be blasphemous to a true believer. Yet not thinking in such terms would prevent a researcher from measuring the effectiveness of prayer in a randomized controlled trial because the method of evaluation requires one to think about prayer as if it were a quantifiable physical intervention. In my view, we ought to abandon the whole idea of trying to study prayer in this way, on these grounds alone.

Assuming that one were to construe prayer as a sort of physical force or energy and that one could assign patients to receive intercessory prayer at random, how would one actually go about measuring the quantity, quality, intensity, frequency, volume, and duration of prayer? Does one minute of centering prayer equal three minutes of rote recitation? In the experiment of Sicher et al., for example, persons praying for the experimental group consisted of Christians, Jews, Buddhists, Native Americans, shamanists, and graduates of schools of bioenergetic and meditative healing. Do the prayers of ten Christians equal the prayers of one highly practiced Buddhist monk? As Chibnall, Jeral, and Cerullo have argued, there is no "construct validity" for prayer as an intervention.[3] What, exactly, is the "substance" that is being delivered to the patients in these studies? If one cannot quantify the intervention in an experiment, one cannot infer a cause-and-effect relationship with a quantifiable outcome.

Outcome Measurements

Furthermore, there are problems with measurements used to assess the outcomes of these studies. Two of the three studies that reported a positive effect of intercessory prayer did so on the basis of statistically significant changes in outcome scales. These scales took account of a variety of outcomes of intensive care, such as whether the patient needed a catheter to measure blood pressure in the lung (a Swan-Ganz catheter) or whether the patient needed to be placed on a ventilator. The measurement scales assigned these and other outcomes a certain number of points and summed them into a global measure of outcome. In the Byrd study, there was a statistically significant positive effect in only six of the twenty-six measured individual items. Importantly, there was no difference in mortality between the groups. Harris et al. measured thirty-three endpoints, and only one was individually statistically significant. Again, importantly, mortality was the same whether patients were prayed for or not. In the third positive study, by Sicher et al., six of eleven endpoints were positive—mostly hospitalization and outpatient visit rates. Neither CD4+ cell counts nor mortality was associated with prayer.

The approach of measuring multiple endpoints raises a complicated methodological problem. When one measures many endpoints, one expects a small number of them to be "statistically significant" at random. Thus, having a few outcomes that are positive is no "proof" of the effectiveness of an intervention. Researchers can circumvent this problem in several ways. One would be to do a Bonferroni correction, which essentially raises the threshold for calling a statistical result "significant." In all three of these positive studies, given the large number of endpoints, if one were to do a Bonferroni correction, the results would all be "negative." The authors of these studies elected not to use Bonferroni-corrected data to deal with the problem of multiple endpoints.

Another way to circumvent these statistical problems would be to do a multivariable analysis, in which all variables are considered together in a statistical method that can balance out random differences, separating true effects from background "noise." Harris et al. did not do this multivariable analysis. Byrd states that such analysis was done but provides no description of the multivariable statistical method used or any data on the actual results of this analysis, except to report that it was "positive"—so we have no way to evaluate this claim scientifically. Sicher et al. are to be commended for doing a multivariable analysis, but they used a nonstandard technique that also attempts to correct for the fact that many of their outcome variables are likely to be correlated with each other. Problems that arise in multivariable analysis when the endpoints are all correlated with each other are referred to as "confounding" and "multi-colinearity." For example, two of the positive endpoints in the study by Sicher et al.—the number of hospitalizations and total hospital days—are likely to be highly correlated with each other. This correlation makes multivariable statistical testing difficult to interpret. Nonetheless, Sicher et al. were at least aware of these problems and did try to account for them, even if their accounting was inadequate.

The third method for dealing with multiple outcome measures is to put all the variables together into what is called a "scale." The studies by Byrd and by Harris et al. used this method. Making an outcome scale is not as simple, however, as just sitting back in a chair and listing all the things that could go right or wrong, giving each a point, and adding them up. In good outcomes research, one must carefully assess the scale and develop each item ahead of time. This step usually is done in separate studies before the study of interest is undertaken. There are many questions to ask about scales. Who says which items are important to include on the scale and how should they be weighted? Patients? Outside experts? General practitioners? Furthermore, one ought to evaluate the scale's statistical properties. Do changes in one item tend to go with changes in all the others, so that it forms a true scale ("internal consistency" or "reliability")? Are there multiple subscales within the scale ("factor analysis")? Has the scale been used before by others, so that one study can be compared with another? Is the scale "sensitive" to differences in the underlying health of the patients? Is it "responsive" to interventions? Neither Byrd nor Harris et al. did any of these things.

Notably, the negative study by Walker and colleagues measured a single outcome—self-reported alcohol consumption—in a commonly used and rigorously validated single-item measure called "Standard Drinking Units." The two positive intensive care unit studies used non-validated, idiosyncratic outcome scales, which makes the results scientifically suspect. In addition, when Harris et al. analyzed their data with the scale used in the Byrd study, their results were negative. Thus, we say that they "failed to replicate" the findings of Byrd—making the putatively positive results in both studies suspect.

Miscellaneous Scientific Problems

Sample size also is an issue in these studies. Small studies are more prone to error, and overly large studies can make even very trivial differences statistically significant. The most methodologically sound studies—by Walker et al. and Sicher et al.—were very small, enrolling forty patients each. The studies by Byrd and by Harris et al. included adequate numbers—hundreds of patients—but were the most methodologically suspect, as I note above.

Finally, one must evaluate these studies for other sources of bias. Data analysis and interpretation can be influenced by the underlying beliefs of the sponsors as well as the investigators. The studies by Byrd and by Harris et al. do not mention grant support. The study by Walker et al. was partially supported by funding from the National Institutes of Health (NIH). The study by Sicher et al. was funded by three sources: the Sausolito Consciousness Research Laboratory, the Institute of Noetic Sciences, and the Parapsychology Foundation. These organizations all promote belief in "mind over matter" phenomena. Before accepting such results as true, one would hope that similar studies funded by more neutral groups would attempt to replicate these findings.

On the basis of these criticisms, I find the empirical studies of the efficacy of intercessory prayer deeply scientifically flawed. There is no good scientific evidence to accept that they have proven that prayer is a medically "efficacious" treatment. Many of my criticisms suggest that better science cannot overcome these problems. Given the inherently insurmountable problems with randomization and the quantification and characterization of prayer, conducting adequate scientific studies of this type among human beings simply would be impossible.

Moral Critique

Beyond the scientific issues, however, the idea of conducting studies on the efficacy of intercessory prayer also poses a significant moral problem for believers. If one believes in God and the power of prayer, engaging in a study in which one intentionally identifies individuals from whom one will withhold prayer seems immoral. If Christ commanded that Christians should pray even for their persecutors (Matt. 5:44), ought Christian researchers not at least pray for their ill research subjects? If one believes in prayer, how could one justify randomizing patients with the intention of withholding prayer from half of them? A believing person should find as many moral problems with a study that chooses some patients not to be prayed for as with a study in a developing country that chooses some pregnant patients not to receive anti-AIDS drugs even with the full knowledge that such drugs prevent perinatal transmission of AIDS in developed countries.[4]

Theological Critique

One also can raise many general theological critiques about randomized trials of intercessory prayer at a distance. The first problem is that these studies invert what ought to be the believer's understanding of the very structure of the universe. By putting God to the test of science, these studies, in effect, make empirical science the arbiter of truth. This ap-

proach implies that the experimenter's faith in science is greater than
the experimenter's faith in God. Amplifying this point, Chibnall, Jeral,
and Cerullo note that the statistical techniques on which experimental
science depends demand that one begin with the "null hypothesis,"
which could be stated in these studies as, "Given the starting belief that
prayer does not work, how likely would the observed results be?" This
question is an odd starting point for a person of faith.

Second, as Cohen et al. have observed, these studies tend to suggest
that the physician is controlling God. Authentic faith, however, demands acknowledgment that God is in control. Thus, these experiments suggest to me the sin of Simon Magus (Acts 8:9–24). Simon—a
magician, even though he had been baptized a Christian—offered the
disciples money to obtain the power of conveying the Holy Spirit by the
laying on of hands. Although one can learn many lessons from this
story, I believe the most fundamental point is not so much that Simon
Magus wanted to pay for this power as that he wanted to control the
Holy Spirit. He wanted to own the Holy Spirit and manipulate the Holy
Spirit at will. He wanted to reduce God to magic and to conjure God's
action and command a power that properly was only God's. At least for
a believing Christian, trying to control or manipulate God's power, even
for a good purpose such as healing, is always a sin against the Spirit.
God is not another implement in the doctor's black bag. God is not
another nostrum in the pharmacopoeia. To think of prayer in this way
is to commit the sin of Simon Magus.

Third, the presuppositions of these studies lead one to theologically
dangerous beliefs about patients who pray for healing and are not
healed. Is one to suppose that God is absent from those who are not
healed? Should one question the purity, intensity, sincerity, quantity, or
duration of these patients' prayers or of those who prayed for them?
From the point of view of true faith, God is never absent from persons
who seek him with a sincere heart. Patients whose prayers for healing
are not answered with healing should not be made to feel guilty; they
must find a way to understand the mysteries with which Christ grappled
at Gethsemane. "Not what I want, but what you want" (Mark 14:36).

Finally, one must consider the theological oddities to which one is committed by consideration of the endpoints in these studies. None of the three positive studies showed an effect on mortality. Does anyone who believes in God and also believes that these studies have proven the efficacy of intercessory prayer honestly believe that God cares enough to reduce the number of Swan-Ganz catheters that are placed in patients who have been prayed for but does not care enough to make more of them survive? This reasoning seems completely absurd.

Misplaced Scientific Critiques

The harshness of my critique of these studies of intercessory prayer at a distance should not be overinterpreted. I obviously believe that spirituality has an important role in health care. In chapter 8 I lay out an explicit program of scientific study of the relationship between spirituality and health. I caution about the limited value of such studies, but I do not dismiss the scientific study of spirituality and health altogether. My critique in this chapter only explains why we should greet one particular set of studies with deep scientific and theological skepticism.

Therefore, I think the scientific critiques offered by Richard Sloan and his colleagues have mistakenly "thrown the baby out with the bathwater."[5] For instance, they have included the numerous studies that have shown an association between church attendance and longevity in their scathing scientific critiques.[6] Although I agree in large measure with their critique of the prayer-at-a-distance studies, their critiques of large epidemiological studies that have shown an association between religious service attendance and longevity are overdrawn at best. The fact that some types of scientific studies about spirituality and health care are scientifically flawed does not imply that all scientific studies of this subject are flawed.

Studies showing that people who attend religious services regularly live longer are convincing and have been carefully carried out. They have involved large numbers of patients followed over decades in various geographic locations. They all roughly agree on the magnitude of the effect. They have controlled for potentially confounding factors such as lower drug, alcohol, and tobacco use among religious service attendees. They have controlled for the fact that sick patients are less likely to attend religious services and therefore are more likely to die. They have controlled for diet, exercise, and high blood pressure. Even after accounting for all of these factors, these studies find that persons who attend religious services regularly live longer. Sloan and his colleagues seem so upset with the implications that have been drawn from these studies that they have tried to denigrate their scientific validity. This attitude is unfair, as well as scientifically disingenuous.

The implications one draws from these studies, of course, constitute an altogether different matter from accepting their results as true. People who attend religious services regularly might live longer because of many factors that may be associated with worshipping behavior. Their religious communities might provide them with a form of social support. Meditation or prayer might affect their immune systems and blood pressure. They might receive from religion a source of hope and a sense of discipline that makes them more likely to be compliant with medications. These or a variety of other factors might mediate the effects of religion on health. Faith would be unnecessary for any of these secondary causes. Yet one must admit that religions tend to give people all of them, as one package deal. I believe that these studies have established a clear association between religious service attendance and longevity. Sloan and his colleagues can accept this conclusion as true without accepting that God is somehow "zapping" persons who go to church or temple and making them healthier.

Sloan and his colleagues argue that interpreting either the prayer-at-a-distance studies or the studies about longevity and religious service attendance as a license for the physician to encourage religious service attendance as a preventive or therapeutic intervention is morally problematic. I agree, and I have more to say about this point in chapter 10. Rejection of the implications that some observers are drawing from these studies does not mean, however, that the studies are scientifically flawed. Such a critique goes too far.

Conclusion

Although many avenues of scientific investigation into the role that spirituality and religion can play in health care are valid and interesting, randomized controlled trials of the effects of intercessory prayer at a distance are deeply flawed—scientifically, morally, and theologically. If one were to conduct enough of these studies and use appropriate endpoints, the outcomes, on average, probably would be the same for both the experimental and the control groups. If God "makes his sun rise on the evil and the good, and sends rain on the righteous and the unrighteous" (Matt. 5:45), one should not expect any different result. Prayer is not about commanding God or asserting one's own will over God's. It is not about magically changing the future. I pray for every one of my patients, but the results are God's business, not mine. The results are part of "the plan of the mystery hidden for ages in God who created all things" (Eph. 3:9). For orthodox Christians, true prayer enables the final, total surrender of one's whole being; in this surrender, which culminates in death, one's life becomes "hidden with Christ in God" (Col. 3:3). For a person of faith, no other outcome really matters.

Notes

1. Randolph C. Byrd, "Positive Therapeutic Effects of Intercessory Prayer in a Coronary Care Unit Population," *Southern Medical Journal* 81 (1988): 826–29; William S. Harris, Manohar Gowda, Jerry W. Kolb, Christopher P. Strychacz, James L. Vacek, Phillip G. Jones, Alan Forker, James H. O'Keefe, and Ben D. McCallister, "A Randomized, Controlled Trial of the Effects of Remote, Intercessory Prayer on Outcomes in Patients Admitted to the Coronary Care Unit," *Archives of Internal Medicine* 159 (1999): 2273–78; Fred Sicher, Elisabeth Targ, Dan Moore, and Helene S. Smith, "A Randomized Double-Blind Study of the Effect of Distant Healing in a Population with Advanced AIDS: Report of a Small Scale Study," *Western Journal of Medicine* 169 (1998): 365–63; Scott R. Walker, J. Scott Tonigan, William R. Miller, Stephen Comer, and Linda Kahlich, "Intercessory Prayer in the Treatment of Alcohol Abuse and Dependence: A Pilot Investigation," *Alternative Therapies in Health and Medicine* 3 (November 1997): 79–86.

2. Cynthia B. Cohen, Sondra E. Wheeler, David A. Scott, Barbara Springer Edwards, and Patricia Lusk, "Prayer as Therapy: A Challenge to Both Religious Belief

and Professional Ethics," Anglican Working Group in Bioethics, *Hastings Center Report* 30 (May–June 2000): 40–47; John A. Astin, Elaine Harkness, and Edzard Ernst, "The Efficacy of 'Distant Healing': A Systematic Review of Randomized Trials," *Annals of Internal Medicine* 132 (2000): 903–10.

3. John T. Chibnall, Joseph M. Jeral, and Michael A. Cerullo, "Experiments on Distant Intercessory Prayer: God, Science, and the Lesson of Massah," *Archives of Internal Medicine* 161 (2001): 2529–36.

4. Peter Lurie and Sheldon M. Wolfe, "Unethical Trials of Interventions to Reduce Perinatal Transmission of the Human Immunodeficiency Virus in Developing Countries," *New England Journal of Medicine* 337 (1997): 853–56.

5. Richard P. Sloan, Emilia Bagiella, Larry VandeCreek, Margot Hover, Carlo Casalone, Trudi Jipnu Hirsch, Yusuf Hasan, Ralph Kreeger, and Peter Poulos, "Should Physicians Prescribe Religious Activities?" *New England Journal of Medicine* 342 (2000): 1913–16; Richard P. Sloan, Emilia Bagiella, and Tia Powell, "Religion, Spirituality, and Medicine," *Lancet* 353 (1999): 664–67.

6. See, for instance, Robert A. Hummer, Richard G. Rogers, Charles B. Nam, and Christopher G. Ellison, "Religious Involvement and U.S. Adult Mortality," *Demography* 36 (1999): 273–85; Harold G. Koenig, Judith C. Hays, David B. Larson, Linda K. George, Harvey J. Cohen, Michael E. McCullough, Keith G. Meador, and Dan G. Blazer, "Does Religious Attendance Prolong Survival? A Six-Year Follow-Up Study of 3,968 Older Adults," *Journal of Gerontology*, Series A, 54, no. 7 (1999): M370–76; J. LeBron McBride, Gary Arthur, Robin Brooks, and Lloyd Pilkington, "The Relationship between a Patient's Spirituality and Health Experiences," *Family Medicine* 30 (1998): 122–26; Douglas Oman and Dwayne Reed, "Religion and Mortality among the Community-Dwelling Elderly," *American Journal of Public Health* 88 (1998): 1469–75; William J. Strawbridge, Richard D. Cohen, Sara J. Shema, and George A. Kaplan, "Frequent Attendance at Religious Services and Mortality over 28 Years," *American Journal of Public Health* 87 (1997): 957–61.

Is There a Moral Obligation to Address the Spiritual Needs of Patients?

Having discussed the philosophical, existential, and historical basis for spirituality in health care and having critiqued the burgeoning empirical literature about this subject in great detail, I now turn to a critical question: Is it morally permissible for health care professionals to address spiritual issues with their patients? This question is now being taken seriously by American health care. Just a few years ago, outside of a few nursing schools one would have been far more likely to overhear discussions of why scientifically trained health care professionals had a moral duty to refrain from addressing spiritual matters with their patients. More likely, the question simply would have been ignored. In recent years, however—thanks in large measure to an initiative funded by the Templeton Foundation—many medical schools have begun to offer spirituality courses, and the medical literature now regularly features articles on the topic. Yet as I note at the end of chapter 9, many clinicians and academics object vigorously to these trends. Thus, the question of whether allowing clinicians to introduce spirituality into their relationships with patients is morally permissible is a lively topic of debate.[1]

I intend to push the limits of this question further. I explore not just whether interested health care professionals should be *permitted* to attend to the spiritual needs of their patients (rather than banning such conversations) but whether there is a moral *obligation* for all health care professionals to attend to their patients' spiritual needs. Given my harsh criticisms of some of the empirical studies about spirituality and health care and some of the invalid implications some observers have drawn from these studies, one might begin to think that I am opposed to this practice. Yet everything I say in Part I of this book would lead one to think that addressing the spiritual needs of patients is essential. In this chapter I explain my own position.

I begin by reviewing some definitions that should now be familiar. Then I argue that the primary moral justification for addressing spiritual issues comes from neither outcomes data nor consumer demand but from the nature of healing. Third, I discuss and rebut arguments against allowing health care professionals to address spiritual issues with their patients. Fourth, I defend what I call the collaborative approach to incorporating spirituality into health care practice. Finally, I say something about the moral limits that ought to constrain the practice of incorporating spirituality into the patient care practices of health care professionals.

Some Definitions

Recall again the distinction I have drawn between spirituality and religion; the two often are confused in debates about the ethics of incorporating spirituality into medical practice. Some objections are based on the presumption that spirituality means religion and that the introduction of religion into the clinical arena necessarily entails proselytizing, offense, and imposition of alien values upon patients. I have defined spirituality, however, as the characteristics and qualities of a person's relationship with the transcendent. This definition suggests that spirituality is different from religion; moreover, by this definition everyone can claim to have a spirituality. This point is especially important because of the large number of Americans who consider themselves "spiritual but not religious."[2] One ought not ignore such persons' needs.

A religion, as I have defined it, is a specific set of beliefs about the transcendent, usually in association with a particular language that describes spiritual experiences and a community that shares key beliefs, as well as certain practices, texts, rituals, and teachings. Although not everyone has a religion, most people give expression to their spirituality through a religion.

Moreover, as I also point out in chapter 2, because every human personality is unique, every human relationship with the transcendent also is unique. Only individual persons can apprehend, question, and live lives that engage the transcendent.

Because this chapter is about the ethics of addressing spirituality in health care, I also must define what I mean by *ethics*. Ethics is systematic, critical, reasoned evaluation and justification of notions of right and wrong, good and evil, and the kinds of persons we ought, or ought not, strive to become. Ethics begins whenever people question their own moral positions or those of others by asking "Why is that right? Why is that wrong? What's good about this? What's bad about that?" The activities of ethics entail justifying one's positions and making convincing arguments.

Many people are skeptical about the moral footing that underlies the introduction of spirituality into health care, so asking whether this activity is a morally good or bad thing is by no means trivial. Moreover, there is a distinction between saying that doing something is morally permissible (i.e., that it is morally optional) and saying that there is a moral duty to do something (i.e., that one is morally obligated to do it). The latter is more difficult to establish and, of course, presumes that the former is true. The position I defend is the more difficult one—not only that it is permissible to address spiritual issues in practice but that there is a moral duty for all health care professionals to address spiritual issues with their patients.

What Could Establish Such a Duty?

Proponents have suggested a variety of justifications for introducing spirituality into medicine. In the subsections that follow, I consider two of the most common justifications: data on the relationship between spirituality and health care outcomes and data suggesting that large numbers of patients want their physicians to address their spiritual needs. I find both inadequate.

Outcomes Data

The first argument that has been advanced to establish that there is a duty to address spiritual issues with patients is that regular religious practice seems to be associated with better health care outcomes. Although I have alluded to some of these studies, I have not discussed them in great detail. For example, the Alameda County study showed a 23 percent lower mortality risk for attendees of regular worship services compared with nonattendees after 28 years of follow-up.[3] Other well-controlled and well-designed studies have reached similar conclusions.[4] Some commentators have suggested that these data constitute a warrant for health care professionals to encourage regular church or temple attendance on the part of their patients as a preventive medical measure.[5]

As I discuss briefly in chapter 7, I disagree with that conclusion. My first objection to this line of thought invokes the naturalistic fallacy. These data alone do not add up to a moral mandate to intervene. Not everything that is good for our personal health or the health of the public is morally appropriate to pursue. I return to this moral question and give other reasons at the end of this chapter; the point now is that the only clinical conclusion one can draw from these data is that knowing whether the patient is a regular attendee at worship services might provide useful prognostic information. Patients who attend religious services regularly tend to live longer. I think we can now accept this finding as an established fact. Other moral considerations aside, however, this datum does not provide a *scientific* warrant for a "spiritual intervention" as a form of preventive medicine.[6]

My second objection, which I also discuss briefly in chapter 7, is that these data describe an association between religious service attendance and longevity but do not prove a cause-and-effect relationship.

To prove that going to church *causes* better health, one would need a randomized controlled trial of patients who attend worship services versus those who do not attend worship services (a study that ought not be done, for what I hope are morally obvious reasons). Without such a study, one cannot determine whether the health of persons who had not been attending worship services regularly could be improved by encouraging them to start going to church or temple. The conundrum for the scientific advocate of encouraging regular church or temple attendance to improve health care outcomes is that one can never really obtain the scientific data necessary to prove that the practice works because producing the data that could provide such a moral justification would be immoral.

Thus, better health care outcomes are neither necessary nor sufficient as a moral warrant for introducing spirituality into health care practice. There are also a host of theological arguments about why this sort of thinking is wrong-headed, some of which I raise in chapters 8 and 9. Suffice to say, however, that scientific data about outcomes by themselves are not a moral warrant for spiritual interventions.

Consumer Demand

A second possible moral warrant for introducing spirituality into health care practice is consumer demand. This possibility seems more plausible to Americans. The reason we need to address spiritual issues in practice, according to some observers, is that patients seem to want it. Certainly, surveys suggest that patients want their physicians to address spiritual issues with them; many even want their physicians to pray with them.[7] If clinicians are to practice patient-centered health care, they need to take their patients' desires seriously. I do not believe, however, that this reason is a sufficient moral warrant for introducing spirituality into health care practice. Not everything patients want or desire is morally justifiable for practitioners to do.

Medicine, nursing, and the other health care professions have their own internal moral and intellectual integrity that regularly limits the scope of what practitioners of these professions can do. Good physicians do not give their patients laetrile for cancer or penicillin for viral pharyngitis even if they desire it. The profession also may refuse to allow its practitioners to perform euthanasia, assist in capital punishment, or be party to torture, even if the majority of the population approves of and desires these actions. Individual patient consent is a *necessary* condition for any spiritual discussion initiated by health care practitioners. However, neither data suggesting that large numbers of patients desire spiritual interventions by their physicians nor repeated requests for a spiritual intervention by an individual patient with intact decision-making capacity constitutes a *sufficient* moral warrant. Although patients must request or at least consent to introduction of spiritual issues into their health care, we must still establish why doctors or nurses ought to do so, even if requested.

Spirituality as Intrinsic to Health Care

If neither outcomes nor patient requests are sufficient to justify introducing spiritual issues into the practice of health care, how can one claim a moral warrant do so? I offer a justification that is based on themes I raise in the opening pages of this book. The argument is simple: Health care professionals are justified in attending to the spiritual concerns of patients because spirituality is *intrinsic* to the practice of the health care professions. The purgation of spirituality from Western health care practice that began slowly during the Renaissance and accelerated sharply during the last half of the twentieth century has been an historical anomaly and a moral mistake.

Spirituality is integral to health care practice. As I argue throughout this book, illness invariably raises a trio of transcendent questions—of meaning, of value, and of relationship. Body and soul cannot be so neatly disentangled as a dualistic, Cartesian approach to health care pretends. Patients are not just bodies—matter and extension. Patients are first and foremost *persons*. Persons are oriented to ask transcendent questions. When a person is ill or dying, he or she asks, "Is there any meaning in my suffering? Do I have any dignity or worth? Is my value to be found only in my social contribution, now limited by my bodily condition? How does this affect my relationships with others? Upon whom can I depend? Can I achieve reconciliation with my loved ones before I die?"

These questions are spiritual. They arise for people of all faiths and for people of no faith. Illness occasions such questions—and science cannot answer them.

The better medical technology has become, the more alienated and frightened patients have become. This phenomenon is not an inevitable tradeoff that people must make as medical science progresses. It is a mistake. Health care that fixes bodies as if they were machines but ignores the transcendent questions that are integral to the personal experience of sickness and death is no longer a healing art. Despiritualized medicine is mistaken in its self-identity.

Regardless of outcomes, spiritual issues are an intrinsic part of health care. The spiritual transcends outcomes. Hence, although debating about whether going to church or temple will prevent myocardial infarctions might be interesting, such debates ultimately are irrelevant to the question. The spiritual issues are already there. All one needs to do is to ask one's patients whether they would like to talk about them.

What Gives Health Care Professionals the Warrant to Address Spiritual Issues?

Even if what I argue is true—that spiritual issues are intrinsic to the experience of illness—this analysis still doesn't quite add up to a warrant for health care professionals to intervene. Why shouldn't this kind of intervention be left to clergy, family, and friends? What gives physicians, nurses, psychologists, and other health care professionals the warrant to address spiritual issues in practice?

Perhaps this question ought to be rephrased. Perhaps what we ought to ask is what gives health care professionals a moral warrant to offer healing in the first place. This question is seldom asked, but it certainly is important. By what moral authority do health professionals render living human persons unconscious and then proceed to stick their fingers into their livers and brains? Consider, for a moment, the fact that there was health care for countless centuries before anything doctors did actually worked. Hence, the moral warrant to practice the healing arts cannot be based on outcomes. What, then, gives doctors, nurses, and other health care professionals a moral warrant to heal?

Pellegrino grounds the moral warrant to heal in what he has called the fact of illness and the act of profession.[8] By the fact of illness he means the patient's predicament—vulnerable, frightened, and unable to help himself or herself. True, the body does often regenerate itself. When it does not, however, one needs the assistance of persons who possess specialized knowledge and skills. Some of their expertise effects cures, some of it ameliorates symptoms, and some of it merely provides diagnostic and prognostic information, but all of it should be provided in a caring and compassionate manner. There is a marked imbalance in freedom, knowledge, and power between persons who are ill and those with a warrant to heal. The only recourse a patient ever has is to trust someone else to help. We all have a stake in this matter. All of us are potential patients.

The trusted other on whom the patient must depend has a social sanction to offer help. That person acquires knowledge and skills through specialized study and training in nursing, medicine, and the other health professions. The practitioner earns the patient's trust through what Pellegrino has called the act of profession. Chapter 6, on the meaning of oath-taking, in some ways, can be interpreted as a spiritual and moral discourse on the act of profession. Health professionals take public oaths that they will use their knowledge and skills "for the good of the sick"; that they will "keep them from harm"; that they will do so "to the best of their ability"; and that they will even put aside self-interest for the good of patients.[9] They swear that they can be trusted to do this. This is their act of profession. They publicly profess that they are worthy to be healers.

What patients need is healing. To heal means to restore the whole person to the state of right relationship. This is what health care professionals swear they will do for their patients.

If illness affected bodies only, one could heal simply by fixing bodies. Human illness does not merely affect bodies, however; it affects persons in their entirety. Human beings are more than the sum of their bodily parts. The human form of being is spiritual being—*Homo religiosus.*[10] Human beings are physical entities that are essentially open to the transcendent: oriented to meaning, value, and relationship. As I argue in chapter 8, illness affects human beings as complete entities—in body and in spirit. Therefore, if health care professionals swear to be healers to the best of their ability and judgment, they are negligent if they do not attend to the spiritual needs of patients. If they refuse to attend to these needs, they are not practicing to the best of their ability and judgment. If they are to be true healers of whole persons, they must attend to the needs of patients as whole persons—including their spiritual needs.

Thus, attention to spiritual needs is a moral imperative. It is not simply a moral option—something that ought to be permitted or tolerated. Attention to the spiritual needs of patients is a moral obligation. The only real question is how to put this obligation into practice.

What Are the Objections?

Many reasonable persons have raised serious ethical questions about introducing attention to patients' spiritual concerns into the relationship between health care professionals and their patients. Religion frightens many people. Religion has been abused—used as a cover for evil—from time immemorial. The concerns the critics now express include concerns that spirituality in medicine is irrelevant, might be intrusive, could amount to proselytizing, might offend some patients, could open the door to charlatanism, might increase patients' sense of guilt, or do other psychological harms. Others worry about imposing such an obligation on nonbelieving health care professionals.

These concerns are real and important. In my view, however, all of these concerns can be addressed adequately, and they need not prevent any clinician from addressing the spiritual concerns of patients in the practice of the various health care professions.

Irrelevant?

Saying that spirituality is irrelevant to clinical practice is simply wrong. This position may be the view of a very small number of patients and the view of a somewhat larger number of health care professionals. Most of these objections, however, are based on a reductionistic approach to medicine or mistaken views about the nature of spirituality. If medicine were simply applied science, this view would be correct. Likewise, if spirituality were completely identified with the pseudo-scientific charlatanism that characterizes too much of what has been classified as alternative medicine, this view would be correct. If what I have said about the nature of medicine, the nature of spirituality, and the essential relationship between them is true, however, then saying that spirituality is irrelevant to health care is simply a mistake.

Too Intimate?

Observers sometimes suggest that spirituality is too personal and private to be shared between clinicians and patients. There certainly is reason to be concerned about needless prying into patients' most personal secrets. On the other hand, the surveys I cite above do seem to show that most patients are interested in having clinicians address spiritual issues. As a society, we accept that physicians may appropriately inquire about many very intimate private details of patients' lives, including their sexual histories. These details are relevant to patient care. Clinicians swear to hold such private information in trust—this is what confidentiality means.

Under the view that spirituality is integrally related to health care and is always relevant, ethical concerns about privacy in relation to the spiritual aspect of care ought to be addressed adequately by the general standards of patient confidentiality. Practitioners simply need to be respectful and keep patients' spiritual histories confidential.

Proselytizing

Addressing patients' spiritual concerns ought never be allowed to degenerate into proselytizing. Using the authority of the white coat to try to win converts or, even worse, to make the delivery of health care services conditional upon the patient's profession of some tenet of religious faith is morally reprehensible.

The imbalance in power between physician and patient and the intimate nature of spiritual concerns precludes proselytizing just as this imbalance in power precludes pursuit of sexual relationships between clinicians and patients. On the other hand, just as this imbalance in power never precludes talking to patients about intimate sexual details in an effort to help them, it ought never preclude talking to patients about their spiritual concerns in an effort to help them.

Offense

Some clinicians fear that at least some patients will be offended by questions about their spiritual lives. The risk seems greatest if the patient belongs to some minority religion or professes no religious beliefs.

Surveys have shown, however, that even among patients who have no religious beliefs, half would welcome a respectful inquiry about their spirituality.[11] Furthermore, if one takes the expansive and inclusive view of spirituality I have taken, these questions should not be offensive to anyone. Inquiring about spirituality in such a broad sense ought not offend a person who does not belong to a particular religious community of any sort. Certainly patients might be *surprised* by questions about their spiritual lives coming from a Western, scientifically educated physician at the beginning of the twenty-first century. If the practitioner carefully explains, however, that spiritual questions about meaning, value, and relationship almost always emerge in the course of illness; that these questions really are spiritual; and that most patients in surveys want clinicians to address these matters, and if the practitioner were to reassure all patients that they are free to defer or decline such discussions, this inquiry should not be offensive.

If a patient were offended by an inquiry about spirituality, conducted in the careful manner I describe, the problem would seem to rest with the patient, not the clinician. As a last resort, if such explanations prove unsatisfactory the patient should always be assured that he or she is free to change physicians.

Charlatanism

There is real concern that all manner of horrific charlatanism will be introduced into health care practice under the guise of "spirituality." I agree fully that this concern is real. Much of the success of Western medicine has been a result of the fact that it has successfully distanced itself from sorcery and alchemy. Patients often are harmed by unproven therapies. The crusade against the "patent medicines" that were foisted on patients at the turn of the twentieth century successfully protected patients from this charlatanism. Recently we were reminded of the potential for alternative medicines to harm patients when L-tryptophan—an alternative, "natural" medicine for sleep, regulated as a food, not a drug—caused an epidemic of eosinophilia-myalgia syndrome.[12]

Nonetheless, medicine ought to be careful not to throw the baby out with the bath water. Alternative treatments ought to be studied scientifically. After all, foxglove, nightshade, and cinchona bark have all proven to be important herbal remedies, from which active ingredients such as digitoxin, belladonna alkaloid, and quinine, respectively, have been purified. In addition, simple respect for the great spiritual traditions of Hinduism, Confucianism, Buddhism, Islam, Judaism, and all the many Christian traditions ought to preclude any attempt to brand all spirituality with the broad label "charlatanism." There is a wide ethical difference between asking patients what role spirituality and religion play in their lives, on one hand, and, on the other hand, offering oneself as a "spiritual healer" who (for a small price) can channel healing energies into patients' tumors by using a special program of secret chants and herbs.

More careful philosophical or theological work on the differences between genuine spirituality and charlatanism would be useful. This research would be an important academic project. At first pass, however, the differences are clear enough to most people of common sense that medicine can effectively promote inclusion of spirituality in practice while avoiding the trap of promoting charlatanism.

Potential Harm to Patients

There is genuine concern that having clinicians talk to patients about spirituality will result in increased patient guilt or other psychological harms. Two groups of patients might be adversely affected. The first group would be patients who profess no spiritual or religious beliefs or practices. Inquiries about their spirituality might make them feel guilty about the fact that they are not particularly religious and might even lead some to believe that they are being punished by God. Others among these patients might fear that the clinician who asked this question might think less of them if they are not religious.

The second group of patients who might be harmed would be religious patients who pray and pray and still become progressively sicker. They might feel guilty that they had not prayed hard enough or had not believed with sufficient fervor. A physician inquiry might exacerbate that guilt.

Much of the basis for these concerns melts away, however, if one takes the position that health outcomes should not be the primary focus of spirituality in medicine. This perspective might be instructive and salubrious for medicine today. Spirituality might represent a potential cure for the new syndrome of "outcomes madness" that is gripping health care. Outcomes and efficiency are the concerns of engineers. Repentance, reconciliation, wonder, awe, gratitude, worship, hope, dignity, meaning, and love are the concerns of *Homo religiosus*.

If one's concerns in addressing the spiritual needs of patients are repentance, reconciliation, wonder, awe, gratitude, worship, hope, dignity, meaning, and love, these needs will always be relevant to every patient, whether the patient is cured or dies. Success and failure, from a spiritual perspective, are not measured in terms of quality-adjusted life-years. As the Christian scriptures say, "For if we live, we live for the Lord, and if we die, we die for the Lord; so then, whether we live or die, we are the Lord's" (Rom. 14:8). From a theological perspective, God is not absent from patients who fare poorly in a biomedical sense. God is not present only to those who fare well. God is with *all* patients. This perspective would provide a healthier foundation for addressing the spiritual concerns of patients without inducing guilt among those who do not recover.

This attitude, however, might not completely allay concerns that patients who do not consider themselves religious could be made to feel guilty. This concern would need to be overcome by promoting the broad approach to spirituality that I present here, rather than one based on narrower denominational concerns. Questions of meaning, value, and relationship arise for patients who are not religious as well. Nevertheless, one can imagine encountering a patient who has completely neglected questions of meaning, value, and relationship in his or her life. Such a patient might feel guilty about these personal failures if asked. If a single question from a physician induces serious guilt in such a patient, however, the patient probably needed to address the issue anyway. It probably had been bubbling near the surface of the patient's conscious attention well before the physician's inquiry.

One also should bear in mind that some guilt is healthy. All human beings ought to be able to recognize their faults and failings and be prepared to change for the better. This kind of guilt would seem to be a prerequisite for the deepest kind of spiritual healing. Hence, it is far from clear how a polite but well-placed question that brings such issues into the patient's consciousness would be a bad thing. If a simple inquiry from a physician could ignite concern for these questions in that person's life, this concern would not be an untoward result, even if it were potentially painful for the patient.

This kind of inquiry must be done skillfully, however. A health care professional who addresses spiritual issues in the setting of the clinician-patient relationship constantly ought to reassure the patient, through words and actions, that lack of interest in the spiritual aspects of life would never limit the clinician's respect for that patient or affect the biomedical aspects of that patient's care in any way. Furthermore, one should be aware that substantial numbers of patients already are experiencing unhealthy religious guilt, believing that their illness is a punishment from God.[13] The opportunity to relieve patients of this guilt presents itself only if questions about spirituality are asked in the clinical setting, the problem is identified, and appropriate interventions are undertaken.

Finally, one must be able to recognize spiritual crises that require the intervention of chaplains or the patient's own clergy and be prepared to make a referral. If the patient's guilt is pathological, one may need to refer to a mental health professional to diagnose and treat depression or some other psychiatric syndrome. Sometimes the distinction between healthy religious stress that can lead to personal growth and pathological conditions is not obvious. Clinicians need to know their limits and when to refer to practitioners with greater expertise in these areas.

What about Nonbelieving Practitioners?

Some atheist or agnostic practitioners might be stunned by the idea that anyone would argue that they have a duty to address the spiritual concerns of their patients. This duty seems to be an imposition upon them. If one understands spirituality in the broad way I have been using the term, however, this obligation should not be a problem after all. Questions of meaning, value, and relationship are important from a purely humanistic perspective even if one denies that there is a God.

Nevertheless, some of these practitioners might not be satisfied with such a response. For some, the word *spirituality* simply cannot be disentangled from religion.[14] Thus, forcing a nonreligious practitioner into making inquiries about patient spirituality might be tantamount to forcing that person to be disingenuous. Such a situation would be a serious moral problem—alienating a person from deeply held personal beliefs.

Even this objection will not hold up, however, under careful scrutiny. Respect for patients as whole persons requires practitioners to be concerned about their patients' concerns, even if the practitioner is morally opposed to the patient's beliefs and practices. Inquiries or expressions of concern should not be taken as endorsement or support of the patient's beliefs and practices, and one can speak carefully to avoid any implication of such an endorsement. For example, if one is morally opposed to abortion and one's patient has just had an abortion, asking, "How did the procedure go?" is not the same as saying, "I have no moral opposition to abortion." Likewise, a nonreligious practitioner can even say explicitly, "I am not a religious person. I do care about you as a person, however, and I know that Islam is important to you. Given how sick you are, I'd like to know if there are any spiritual or religious issues that your illness raises for you. If so, is there any way I can help to facilitate or accommodate your spiritual or religious needs right now?"

How Should Spirituality Be Addressed in the Health Care Setting?

If one grants that spirituality ought to be addressed in the clinical setting and that the counterarguments are not sufficient to refute this position, the remaining question is: How should this interaction be concretely structured? Who should address these issues? What shape should it take?

There are three possible models for addressing spiritual concerns in the clinical setting. I call them the Doctor–Priest Model, the Parallel Track Model, and the Collaborative Ministry Model. I argue in favor of the Collaborative Ministry Model.

The Doctor–Priest Model

Health care professionals might want to return to a sort of shamanism in which the spiritual concerns of patients in the health care setting were the exclusive concern of the health care professionals them-selves—physicians, nurses, and psychologists. After all, if spiritual concerns are integral to health care, logic apparently would dictate that health care professionals should do the work themselves. This is the Doctor–Priest Model. I do not think this arrangement is the wisest, however. Although a complete break between health care and spirituality may be an historical anomaly and a clinical mistake, maintaining some separation between health care and spirituality would be salubrious.

There are several reasons for this position. First, there are issues of expertise to consider. Physicians, nurses, psychologists, and other health care professionals cannot justly claim that they have any spiritual expertise by virtue of their professional training per se. Few have been formally trained as spiritual counselors. I take the Hippocratic Oath's curious clause that one should "never use the knife but should defer to those skilled in that art" as a symbolic pledge not to overstep one's expertise. We live in an age of specialization unknown in earlier cultures in which shamanism developed. Physicians, nurses, and others could do a great deal of damage in trying to take on as well the role of rabbi, imam, or pastor.

One also should bear in mind that my main argument in this chapter is one in favor of having clinicians address the spiritual concerns of patients. Yet by *addressing* I do not mean that doctors and nurses are the ones who need to make the necessary spiritual interventions. Making a diagnosis of lymphoma, for example, does not imply that one is qualified to treat lymphoproliferative malignancies: That is why there is such a thing as a referral.

Second, there are boundary issues to consider. A patient might wish to tell a doctor or nurse certain things that he or she might not want to tell a chaplain, and vice versa. Shared prayer, for instance, is a very intimate event. I am not convinced that it should be a regular occurrence between health care professionals and patients. At the right time and the right place with the right parties, there are moments when it is exactly the proper thing to do. Knowing when is a matter of clinical judgment.

Making it routine is a different matter, however. Certainly, some practitioners advertise that they pray with all their patients, and they attract a self-selected group of patients who very much want prayer as part of their treatment. This practice does not seem problematic. It is far from clear, however, that prayer with patients should be the norm for medical or nursing practice. Many patients could become confused if health care professionals were to become their spiritual counselors. Suppose that a patient contracts gonorrhea after he has had sex with a prostitute. If he discloses this fact to his Doctor–Priest, he might be unclear about whether he is confessing his sins or merely disclosing sensitive but relevant medical information. Although the words might be the same in both situations, the difference in meaning between a confession and a sexual history would depend on the forum.

A wise practitioner will recognize that the biological and the spiritual are simply two aspects of the same experience for the patient, and healing the patient depends on successful restoration of all the disruptions that illness brings on each human being. Arguing that the physician needs to be the one who heals both the biological and the spiritual aspects of the patient's condition is another matter altogether, however.

Finally, there is the danger of opening the door to charlatanism. One way to safeguard against this danger is to carefully circumscribe the aspects of patients' spiritual lives that physicians ought to address directly. This constraint would inhibit charlatanism, as well as any sort of antiscientific bias that could be detrimental to patients and would be inconsistent with a genuine, mature spirituality in health care.

The cautious restrictions I am advocating should not be misunderstood. I am arguing *for* having health care professionals explore spiritual issues with patients. I am advocating only that health care professionals ought not, as a general rule, also be the practitioners of spiritual healing in its most explicit sense. Again, this argument does not mean that—with the right words, the right attitudes, and the right gestures—doctors, nurses, and other health care professionals could not effect spiritual healing even as they are healing the body. I am only suggesting that, as a general rule, spiritual healing by health care professionals should occur indirectly. If direct intervention seems warranted, referral to persons trained to do so probably is best. In other words, physicians and nurses should not return to being shamans.

The Parallel Track Model

The other model—rarely explicitly promulgated but probably the most common practice today—can be called the Parallel Track Model. In this model doctors, nurses, and other health care professionals do their thing, and chaplains do theirs. In this model, health care professionals never inquire about the spiritual needs of the patients and never communicate with chaplains or clergy, except in extreme circumstances. Doctors and nurses take care of the physical and perhaps the psychological. At the same time, the pastoral care department might be very active, or the patient's own clergy might visit regularly. Thus, the patient's spiritual needs might be amply addressed, but on a parallel track.

There are several problems with this approach. First, it symbolizes the false dichotomy between spirituality and medicine that I have taken pains to criticize as anomalous and mistaken. Thus, it continues to lend support to a model of medical practice that is dehumanizing precisely when the rehumanization of medicine is needed. It signals that the personal is unimportant—a sideshow of little consequence to real medicine. Second, it supports the reductionistic philosophy of Foucault's clinic, in which the spiritual is treated like an organ system, with its own specialist (perhaps akin to the role Descartes assigned the pineal gland as the organ of the soul). The fragmentation of health care into multiple sub-subspecialties, with no primary care practitioner to coordinate care and be genuinely concerned about the care of the patient as a whole person, is precisely what stands most in need of remedy in medicine. Subspecialty care, such as cardiology and nephrology, too often is delivered on parallel tracks. Carving out spirituality only compounds these problems. Third, there is a practical issue. If a chaplain sees a patient early in the course of hospitalization and things seem fine, the chaplain might not return unless a referral is made. A hospital might not have a well-developed pastoral care program, and patients might need to rely on their own clergy. If no health care professionals were paying attention to the spiritual needs of patients, however, how would they recognize a genuine spiritual need? How would the patient get the help he or she might need, even in a spiritual crisis? Who would make the referral if all health care professionals thought spirituality were none of their business? Finally, another practical problem with this model is that it could lead to widespread inattention to the spiritual needs of religionless patients. Although such patients might reject the

assistance of clergy, according to my account they still would have genuine spiritual needs. How would these needs be recognized and addressed if the health care professionals did not consider it part of their
jobs to do so? On the whole, then, the Parallel Track Model seems
inadequate.

The Collaborative Model

The Collaborative Model offers the best care for patients. Under this
model, health care professionals and pastoral care professionals would
work collaboratively with patients, as valued members of the health
care team. Health care professionals would learn to recognize the spiritual needs of patients, address them in a simple and basic manner, practice in a way that is deeply respectful of patients' varying spiritualities,
and refer patients to the pastoral care service, the patient's personal
clergy, or perhaps a social worker or yoga instructor, as appropriate.
Likewise, pastoral care members would refer freely when they recognize cognitive difficulties, possible psychiatric problems, or even the
fact that the patient's level of pain is interfering with his or her ability
to concentrate enough to pray.

There are multiple strategies and methods for implementing this
sort of model. In some institutions, clergy members go on rounds with
physicians and nurses on a regular schedule. Increasingly, chaplains
write notes in patients' charts. Chaplains also might take part in multidisciplinary patient care rounds. Physicians occasionally might begin to
ask the patient's permission to stay in the room in respectful silence
while a patient and a chaplain pray. Physicians might learn to cultivate
good working relationships with clergy members in the local area to
whom they might refer their outpatients. Hospice seems to have been
most effective in implementing these strategies and truly integrating
spiritual aspects into the care of dying patients. Spiritual issues arise for
patients long before death, however, and patients would benefit if the
hospice movement's example were made more general in health care
practice.

Genuine ethical issues do arise in this Collaborative Model, but they can be overcome. For example, there is a need for more careful thinking about whether chaplains should write notes in the chart and what they should write if they do. Issues of confidentiality with clergy should take precedence over the otherwise desirable goal of being part of a multidisciplinary team and sharing all patient knowledge freely. Conversely, there may be some things patients want to tell physicians that ought not be disclosed to clergy. More thinking needs to be done about the conditions under which physicians, nurses, or other health care professionals ought to pray with patients. Answering the questions that realization of the Collaborative Model might raise will require sustained, systematic, interdisciplinary reflection. .

Encouraging Patient Religious Practice

I return to one final question about moral limits within this collaborative model that deserves more attention than I have given it: Ought physicians or other health care professionals actively encourage religious practice among their patients because of the associated health benefits? My answer is no.

First, the imbalance in power between health care professionals and patients suggests that one should be very cautious about direct and specific involvement in as intimate and personal a relationship as that between the patient and the transcendent. Such a practice would be analogous to suggesting that unmarried patients ought to marry because married persons have better health outcomes.

Second, this practice would distort the hierarchy of patient goods that health professionals have sworn to uphold. According to Pellegrino and Thomasma's fourfold notion of the patient's good, the good of the patient is an expansive but hierarchical concept.[15] The lowest level of the patient's good is the biomedical good. The next higher level is the good of the patient's choice, followed by the patient's good as a person with intrinsic dignity. The highest level of the patient's good is the ultimate good as the patient sees it—typically described in religious terms.

Suggesting that the patient should seek religion to improve his or her biomedical good would invert that hierarchy of goods—making the lowest level more important than the highest.

Third, encouraging religious belief to serve the patient's bodily health seems odd from a theological perspective. Religion typically is regarded not as an instrumental good but as a good in itself—a difference sometimes called the difference between intrinsic and extrinsic religiosity. If there are health benefits to religiosity, that is a happy coincidence. True love of God, however, does not depend on the health benefits. It might even require a shorter life—as Jesus of Nazareth discovered on Calvary.

Fourth, religious clinicians should be wary of reducing God to a therapeutic nostrum they carry around in their black bag. From a religious perspective, God heals through the clinician, not the other way around.

Finally, as I argue at several points in this book, outcomes are beside the point for a healthy spirituality. Genuine spirituality might even serve as a healthy corrective for the instrumentalist reasoning that so dominates American thinking. The transcendent is always now. The transcendent is to be sought as an end in itself, not as a means to an outcome.

Conclusion

With these caveats and cautions, I restate my thesis: There *is* a moral duty to address spiritual matters in health care. This duty is grounded not in improved health care outcomes or consumer demand but in the nature of illness and healing. This duty must be carried out carefully, avoiding any kind of proselytizing or charlatanism. It cannot be done well on the Parallel Tracks Model. Health professionals have a duty to recognize and elicit patients' spiritual concerns and respect patients' spiritual struggles. Their duty is not to provide spiritual service or counsel on a routine basis, however. The Collaborative Model is preferable to neoshamanism. Clinicians have a duty to help their patients, aided by clergy, in addressing the spiritual issues that arise as a matter of course in the face of illness—the recurring questions of meaning, value, and relationship.

If we are to heal patients as whole persons, we cannot avoid these questions. Learning how to heal this way is one of the great challenges health care faces if the clinic is to experience true rebirth.

Notes

1. Representative articles in favor of incorporating spirituality in medical practice include Bernard Lo, Delaney Ruston, Laura W. Kates, Robert M. Arnold, Cynthia B. Cohen, Kathy Faber-Langendoen, Steven Z. Pantilat, Christina M. Puchalski, Timothy R. Quill, Michael W. Rabow, Simeon Schreiber, Daniel P. Sulmasy, James A. Tulsky, and the Working Group on Religious and Spiritual Issues at the End of Life, "Discussing Religious and Spiritual Issues at the End of Life: A Practical Guide for Physicians," *Journal of the American Medical Association* 287 (2002): 749–54; Steven G. Post, Christina M. Puchalski, and David B. Larson, "Physicians and Patient Spirituality: Professional Boundaries, Competency, and Ethics," *Annals of Internal Medicine* 132 (2000): 578–83. Articles opposing this practice include Richard P. Sloan, Emilia Bagiella, Larry VandeCreek, Margot Hover, Carlo Casalone, Trudi Jipnu Hirsch, Yusuf Hasan, Ralph Kreeger, and Peter Poulos, "Should Physicians Prescribe Religious Activities?" *New England Journal of Medicine* 342 (2000): 1913–16; R. P. Sloan, E. Bagiella, and T. Powell, "Religion, Spirituality, and Medicine," *Lancet* 353 (1999): 664–67; Neil Scheurich, "Reconsidering Spirituality and Medicine," *Academic Medicine* 78 (2003): 356–60.

2. Don Lattin, "Living the Religious Life of None: Growing Numbers Shed Organized Church for Loose Spiritual Sensibility," *San Francisco Chronicle* (December 4, 2003), A1; Barry A. Kosmin and Ergon Mayer, "American Religious Identification Survey, 2001," available at www.gc.cuny.edu/faculty/research_studies.htm#aris_1.

3. William J. Strawbridge, Richard D. Cohen, Sara J. Shema, and George A. Kaplan, "Frequent Attendance at Religious Services and Mortality over 28 Years," *American Journal of Public Health* 87 (1997): 957–61.

4. Robert A. Hummer, Richard G. Rogers, Charles B. Nam, and Christopher G. Ellison, "Religious Involvement and U.S. Adult Mortality," *Demography* 36 (1999): 273–85; Harold G. Koenig, Judith C. Hays, David B. Larson, Linda K. George, Harvey J. Cohen, Michael E. McCullough, Keith G. Meador, and Dan G. Blazer, "Does Religious Attendance Prolong Survival? A Six-Year Follow-Up Study of 3,968 Older Adults," *Journal of Gerontology*, series A 54, no. 7 (1999): M370–76; J. LeBron McBride, Gary Arthur, Robin Brooks, and Lloyd Pilkington, "The Relation-

ship between a Patient's Spirituality and Health Experiences," *Family Medicine* 30 (1998): 122–26; Douglas Oman and Dwayne Reed, "Religion and Mortality among the Community-Dwelling Elderly," *American Journal of Public Health* 88 (1998): 1469–75.

5. Harold G. Koenig, "Should Doctors Prescribe Religion? Interview by Anita J Slomski," *Medical Economics* 77 (January 10, 2000): 144–46, 151, 155; Dale A. Matthews and Connie Clark, *The Faith Factor* (New York: Viking Press, 1998).

6. Daniel P. Sulmasy, "The Ethics of Preventive Medicine," in *Twenty Common Problems: Ethics in Primary Care,* ed. Jeremy Sugarman (New York: McGraw-Hill, 2000), 49–65.

7. These findings are surveyed in Alan B. Astrow and Daniel P. Sulmasy, "Spirituality and the Patient-Physician Relationship," *Journal of the American Medical Association* 291 (2004): 2884. Specific citations on this topic include Timothy P. Daaleman and Donald E. Nease, "Patient Attitudes Regarding Physician Inquiry into Spiritual and Religious Issues," *Journal of Family Practice* 39 (1994): 564–68; John W. Ehman, Barbara B. Ott, Thomas H. Short, Ralph C. Ciampa, and John Hansen-Flaschen, "Do Patients Want Physicians to Inquire about Their Spiritual or Religious Beliefs If They Become Gravely Ill?" *Archives of Internal Medicine* 159 (1999): 1803–6; Dana E. King and Bruce Bushwick, "Beliefs and Attitudes of Hospitalized Patients about Faith Healing and Prayer," *Journal of Family Practice* 39 (1994): 349–52; Charles D. MacLean, Beth Susi, Nancy Phifer, Linda Schultz, Deborah Bynum, Mark Franco, Andria Klioze, Michael Monroe, Joanne Garrett, and Sam Cykert, "Patient Preference for Physician Discussion and Practice of Spirituality," *Journal of General Internal Medicine* 18 (2003): 38–43; Gerard A. Silverstri, Sommer Knittig, James S. Zoller, and Paul J. Nietert, "Importance of Faith on Medical Decisions Regarding Cancer Care," *Journal of Clinical Oncology* 21 (2003): 1379–82; Pamela G. Reed, "Preferences for Spiritually Related Nursing Interventions among Terminally Ill and Non-Terminally Ill Hospitalized Adults and Well Adults," *Applied Nursing Research* 4 (1991): 122–28.

8. Edmund D. Pellegrino, "Toward a Reconstruction of Medical Morality: The Primacy of the Act of Profession and the Fact of Illness," *Journal of Medicine and Philosophy* 4 (1979): 32–56.

9. Quotations are from Ludwig Edelstein, "The Hippocratic Oath: Text, Translation, and Interpretation," in *Ancient Medicine: Selected Papers of Ludwig Edelstein,* ed. Owsei Temkin and C. Lillian Temkin (Baltimore: Johns Hopkins University Press, 1943), 3–63. One of the clearest expressions of the requirement for at least a modicum of altruism among members of a genuine profession is in Abraham Flexner, "Is Social Work a Profession?" *School and Society* 1 (1915): 901–11, which I discuss in detail in chapter 6.

10. Mircea Eliade, *The Sacred and the Profane: The Nature of Religion,* trans. Willard R. Trask (New York: Harcourt, Brace, Jovanovich, 1959), 8–18.

11. Ehman et al., "Do Patients Want Physicians to Inquire about Their Spiritual or Religious Beliefs?"

12. Lee E. Kaufman and Roberta J. Seidman, "L-tryptophan-associated Eosino-philia-Myalgia Syndrome: Perspective of a New Illness," *Rheumatic Diseases Clinics of North America* 17 (May 1991): 427–41.

13. See, for example, Lauris C. Kaldjian, Janes F. Jekel, and Gerald Friedland, "End-of-Life Decisions in HIV-Positive Patients: The Role of Spiritual Beliefs," *AIDS* 12, no. 1 (1998): 103–7, reporting 44 percent of HIV-positive patients with guilt. See also R. N. Eidinger and David V. Schapira, "Cancer Patients' Insight into Their Treatment, Prognosis, and Unconventional Therapies, *Cancer* 53 (1984): 2736–40, which reports that 6.4 percent of cancer patients believed their cancer was a punishment from God. Moreover, this negative religious coping style has been associated with negative health care outcomes; see Kenneth I. Pargament, Harold G. Koenig, Nalini Tarakeshwar, and June Hahn, "Religious Coping Methods as Predictors of Psychological, Physical and Spiritual Outcomes among Medically Ill Elderly Patients: A Two-Year Longitudinal Study," *Journal of Health Psychology* 9 (2004): 713–30.

14. Scheurich, "Reconsidering Spirituality and Medicine."

15. Edmund D. Pellegrino and David C. Thomasma, *For the Patient's Good: The Restoration of Beneficence in Health Care* (New York: Oxford, 1988).

Part III

At the Threshold of Death

In this last section of the book I address spiritual issues that arise in patient care at the close of life. As I state in the Introduction, I do not suggest that spiritual issues arise only as death draws near. Spirituality is not just for persons who are dying. Spirituality runs in a broad and deep channel through health care. Spirituality is always for the living, whether they are healthy or sick, young or old, beginning life or nearing its end. That is why I began this book with general considerations about spirituality and health care.

In the preceding chapters, however, I have skirted the topic of death. I have done so not because I think the topic can or should be avoided. In fact, death pervaded the text—but in an oblique fashion, surfacing only in discussions of finitude and suffering. Yet a book about spirituality and health care cannot avoid a direct confrontation with death. Most persons—if they consider the relationship between spirituality and health care at all—think about spirituality in the setting of death. The spiritual issues that arise at the end of life do not differ from those that arise in acute and chronic illness. Nonetheless, when death looms, the spirit is concentrated as much as the mind. Spiritual issues assume a saliency and intensity in this setting that make it especially useful for clinicians and patients to examine them as they unfold at the close of life. I hope it will be obvious, however, that these issues are relevant to patients with acute nonlethal conditions and chronic conditions as well.

In chapter 11 I treat the topic of miracles. In chapter 12 I offer an overview of spiritual issues in the care of persons who are dying. In chapter 13 I amplify discussion of the particular themes of dignity and reconciliation as portrayed in the play *W;t*. In chapter 14 I tell the story of one patient's spiritual struggles at the end of life (as well as those of her physician).

In addressing spiritual issues in the care of persons who are dying, I draw on many themes raised in preceding chapters, such as suffering, prayer, dignity, and the meaning of healing. These ideas are propadeutic to the task of discussing spirituality at the end of life. In these concluding chapters, I focus on the simple fact that the closer one comes to the edges of life, the more clearly one comes to confront the transcendent.

~~ 11

On Praying for a Cure

Whenever nurses, social workers, or house officers are asked to present a case about spiritual issues in health care practice, they almost always initially choose a case involving a dying patient whose family refuses to authorize a "do not resuscitate" (DNR) order because they are praying for a miraculous cure. These cases often are quite distressing and polarizing. People of real faith pray for cures. They believe God listens to their prayers. They believe God is active in the world. If these propositions are true, persons of a variety of faiths tend to conclude that one must believe that prayer can change a patient's condition by moving God to intervene supernaturally in the world. Some readers might feel that my reluctance to endorse experiments designed to prove the power of prayer indicates a lack of faith on my part—a skeptical modern discomfort with the idea of miracles. Despite my critique of experiments designed to test the healing power of intercessory prayer as a scientific hypothesis, however, I am not a skeptic about prayer, God's concern for human needs, or God's power. I propose a Catholic, Christian understanding of what praying for a cure means. This understanding supports a cautious approach to the idea of scientific studies of the healing power of intercessory prayer, yet requires deeper faith in God than some observers would think.

Many skeptics suppose that modern science excludes miracles. This skepticism presupposes a distinction between the natural (i.e., what can be explained by scientific laws of nature) and the supernatural (i.e., what cannot be explained by scientific laws of nature). The skeptic supposes that everything that happens is natural and can be explained by the laws of nature (at least potentially). Because the skeptic identifies the miraculous with what cannot be explained by the scientific laws of nature, the skeptic concludes that there can be no miracles.

Philosopher and theologian Bernard Lonergan points out that the major flaw in this argument is not so much that it denies the supernatural but that it rests on an archaic view of science.[1] Scientists today understand that the universe is entirely contingent, rather than necessary. What happens in the natural universe is based largely on probabilities; *from a scientific point of view*, things could have been otherwise. Furthermore, our scientific laws are all *ceteris paribus* laws—in other words, "other things being equal, this is true." In this understanding, the distinction between the natural and the supernatural, as the skeptic assumes it is defined, simply disappears. There can be no distinction between that which follows the scientific laws of nature and that which does not because the scientific laws of nature are not *necessary*. The miraculous cannot be defined by a distinction that does not exist.

Perhaps this analysis gives new meaning to the traditional Catholic teaching that God acts through secondary causes.[2] Secondary causation is a term that traditionally has been used to describe how God acts in and through the natural order he has created, not outside of nature and not contrary to the laws of his own creation. It might be logically possible for God to act directly, outside the laws of nature. Certainly, Christians are dogmatically committed to some major instances of primary acts on the part of God, such as the Incarnation and the Resurrection. One need not be constrained, however, by the belief that *miracle* necessarily denotes an event in which God acts outside of nature. Not only are the laws of nature contingent, nature itself is contingent. God is present to all of nature—not merely *in* nature or co-extensive with nature—but necessarily present to a radically contingent universe as the ground of its existence in every place and in every moment. The universe is contingent; God is its only necessity.

Thus understood, God is not present to some patients who are cured because they were successful in appeasing God with their prayers and absent from other patients who were not cured because they failed to pray. God is present to all patients—including those who did not pray and were cured anyway and those who prayed and prayed and prayed and were not cured. Praying or not, cured or not, God is always present. Believing this tenet requires a far more radical faith than believing that God alights on some patients, rarely, with neon lights flashing, *Deus ex machina*, effecting miraculous cures for them, while remaining coldly distant from the rest.

A miracle is not something that scientific laws cannot explain. Indeed, scientific laws cannot explain that there *is* a universe to begin with. The first order of contingency is creation—without God there is no universe to try to explain. The second order of contingency is the very structure of this universe. The laws by which the universe we have come to understand operates are probabilistic, and our scientific explanations therefore are always *ceteris paribus*.

Thus understood, God is not the scientific explanation of last resort. For a religious person, invoking God's name to explain what one cannot explain by science borders on blasphemy. God is not a stopgap for all the *lacunae* in human knowledge. God is the ground of human knowledge.

Worse still is insistence on using science to prove God's power. Thinking this way puts science above God, subjecting God to scientific scrutiny. The Christian scriptures hold that even Jesus was tempted in this way. He resisted, however, quoting Deuteronomy 6:16: "Again it is written, 'Do not put the Lord your God to the test'" (Matt. 4:7). This quote amounts to another explanation of what is theologically wrong with scientific studies that purport to test the efficacy of prayer. Such studies reduce God to a form of scientific explanation; in fact, God is the ground of scientific explanation.

Thus, patients who pray for a cure and are not cured can be liberated from the fear that they have not prayed with sufficient fervor or are unworthy or the conclusion that God must not have answered their prayers. On this understanding, God is not absent from them. Nor should the believer spend time worrying that God has unjustly rewarded nonbelievers or those who do not pray and yet are cured. God, who "makes his sun to rise on the evil and the good, and sends rain on the righteous and the unrighteous" (Matt. 5:45), is absent from neither.

What Does God Hope to Accomplish by Way of Miracles?

For all the stories of miracles in the history of Roman Catholicism, the word "miracle" occurs only eight times in the entire Catechism of the Catholic Church.[3] Six of the eight citations refer to the miracles of Jesus, one to the "miracles of Christ and the saints," and one to the special gifts of the Holy Spirit. Like other charisms of the Holy Spirit, miracles—such as cures from cancer or awakenings from coma—are gifts that, by their very nature, "are oriented toward sanctifying grace and are intended for the common good of the Church" (§ 2003). Orthodox Catholic theology teaches that the purpose of miracles is not to reward the faithful but to upbuild the spiritual life of the whole people of God and to "strengthen faith in the One who does his father's works. . . . they are not intended to satisfy people's curiosity or desire for magic" (§ 548).

The experience of the miraculous is not a matter of God's presence or absence. Christians believe that God is always present to everyone. When one encounters an event that one deems miraculous, what matters is the message, not the event itself. What matters to God is that people see the events of their lives through the eyes of faith. Catholic Christianity teaches that in certain instances, God's Word, which is always trying to break in upon the lives of human beings and reveal God's love for them, does so in a profound way. The circumstances in which this revelation occurs are apt to be unusual—enough to shake one from one's mundane, humdrum existence, self-pity, and narcissistic egotism. These unusual circumstances reveal to people who they are and who God is, in a way that is qualitatively different from all the other moments of worship, ministry, work, family life, or study.

Whenever and wherever this revelation happens—whether one sees a vision on a mountaintop or witnesses the resuscitation of a loved one who had been taken for dead—one often calls these moments "miracles." These burning bush moments (Ex. 3:1–6), Transfiguration moments (Luke 9:28–36), and Lazarus moments (John 11:1–44) have a definite function for every believing person, just as they had in the lives of the first disciples of Jesus. These moments are one's miracles. These moments are qualitatively different from other moments in one's life. If one were writing one's spiritual autobiography, these moments would count as special experiences of God's grace.

This is not to say that God's grace is absent from the other moments of one's life. In a metaphysical sense, God is no more present in these moments than in other moments. Just as God was present with Moses when he stood before Pharaoh and at his side throughout the years of wandering in the desert; just as Jesus was with the first disciples in all the other moments of their lives, not just in those very special moments on Mount Tabor or at a gravesite in Bethany, the faithful today can know that God is always with them as well. He is with them in sickness and in health, in recovery and in death. The task of the faithful is to listen more closely to what God is trying to tell them, so that they know and believe that "whether we live or whether we die, we are the Lord's" (Rom. 14:8).

Praying for Miracles

What, then, is the point of prayer for the sick—of praying for one's own recovery or for that of another? If prayer doesn't seem to change anything, why bother?

Understanding the harmony between the notion of the miraculous that I have sketched out and the notion of petitional prayer requires a healthy understanding of prayer. One simple way to understand the fundamental importance of prayer in Christian living is to note that in contrast to the eight oblique citations in the Catechism about miracles, all of Part IV of the Catechism (seventy-five pages) is devoted to prayer.

Prayer is "the raising of one's mind and heart to God or the requesting of good things from God" (§ 2559). The Catechism calls prayer a "gift" from God to each person (§ 2559), a covenant between God and each person, lived in the heart (§2563–64), and a communion with the Trinity and the saints (§ 2565).

When people pray, they do ask God for good things, however bold and presumptuous this request might seem. In fact, petitional prayer is the simplest, most spontaneous, and often the most heartfelt form of prayer. When we make our needs—or those of others—known to God in prayer, first and foremost "we express awareness of our relationship with God. We are creatures who are not our own beginning, not the masters of adversity, not our own last end" (§ 2929).

In this sense, sincere prayer always "works." The work of prayer is not to force God to bend the future to one's will. The work of prayer is to open oneself to the grace of God, which is always nearer to us than we imagine. The work of prayer is to tell God of one's deepest hopes and fears and to let God flood one's heart. Prayer happens when a woman walks into an intensive care unit, perhaps for the first time in her life; sees her almost unrecognizable husband swollen with saline and tethered to a ventilator; and prays, spontaneously, from the depths of her being, "Oh God, please help him." With this prayer, she offers to God her very vulnerability, her love for her husband, and her recognition of his fragility. She expresses her faith that the Holy Spirit prompts her prayer, her faith that the love of Christ subsumes her love, her faith that the providential power of the Father redeems even this situation. This faith makes her simple, intercessory petition on behalf of her husband the deepest and purest of prayers. When she goes home again at night she prays the same prayer and shares her doubts as well as her faith with God. She cries with Christ, in her own words and in her own voice, "Eloi, Eloi, lema sabachthani" (Mark 15:34). She prays that her children will have the strength to bear seeing their father in such a state. She prays that the Lord will be with the doctors to guide them to do the best they possibly can for her husband. She prays that she might be a source of encouragement to her husband and to her children. To which the church responds: Amen.

This woman is not commanding God. She is not demanding results. She is lifting up her heart and her mind and asking for good things.

That is enough for God, for her husband, and for her. In God's providential plan for this woman and her husband—and in God's time, not hers—her prayers will be answered. The desire she expresses in her prayer and the opening of her heart to God is precisely the point of her prayer.

Prayer always changes things. As Annie Dillard writes, "True prayer surrenders to God; that willing surrender itself changes the situation a jot or two by adding power which God can use."[4]

The fact that a person prays *does* change the situation. The bare fact that prayer has occurred means that the situation is different than it might have been if no one had prayed. The God who is just as present to the future (and the past) as to the present hears that prayer and already has incorporated that prayer, providentially, into the future. From the human perspective, God has changed the situation in response to prayer. How this change appears to God, who is outside of time, only God knows. To a genuine believer, it does not matter. The prayer matters.

If one truly believes in the providential love of God, God's answer is whatever unfolds for us. Prayer calls each person to grapple with life and to find God in the midst of it, whatever it brings. Augustine says that God warns us to be careful about our prayers, so that "no one may think well of himself if his prayer is heard, when he has asked impatiently for what it would be better for him not to receive, and that no one may be cast down and may despair of the divine mercy toward him if his prayer has not been heard when he has, perhaps, asked for something which would bring him more bitterness if he received it, or would cause his downfall if he were ruined by prosperity. In such circumstances, then, we know not what we should pray for as we ought. Hence, if anything befalls us contrary to what we pray for, by bearing it patiently, and giving thanks in all things, we should never doubt that we ought to ask what the will of God intends, and not what we will ourselves."[5]

This is how prayer "works." Prayer is not a matter of magically changing the course of events. Faith commits a person to trust in God and believe that God has a providential plan for each of us. One is free to love or sin, to listen to God or run from God. Certainly, outside of human time, the free choices of human beings already are known to God. Such foreknowledge, however, is not predestination. People do make free choices, and the choices they make do affect their future within the limits of its finitude. The unfolding of one's biological fini-tude, one's sickness and one's health, one's life and one's death, is not something one can completely control, however. The only free choices one ever makes that transcend the limits of one's finite futures are the choices one makes to love. The making of these choices is how prayer changes the world. To pray is to say one loves God and is open to re-ceiving God's love. To pray for the health of another person is to say that one loves that person. Thus, prayer always brings a person one step closer to complete restoration of universal right relationship. Rightly understood, prayer *always* heals.

Notes

1. Bernard J. F. Lonergan, *Method in Theology*, 2nd ed. (New York: Herder and Herder, 1972), 226.
2. Karl Rahner, *Foundations of Christian Faith*, trans. William V. Dych (New York: Crossroad, 1978), 86–89.
3. *Catechism of the Catholic Church* (Liguori, Mo.: Liguori Publications, 1994), § 156, 434, 468, 515, 548, 561, 1335, 2003.
4. Annie Dillard, *For the Time Being* (New York: Vintage, 2000), 169.
5. St. Augustine, "To Proba," no. 130 in *Letters*, vol. 2, trans. Wilfrid Parsons, Fathers of the Church Series, vol. 18 (Washington, D.C.: Catholic University of America Press, 1953), 397.

~~ 12

Healing the Dying

In the final analysis, every dying person who retains the capacity to hear and understand the call of death must face the three important sets of questions I describe in part I of this book: questions of *value*, questions of *meaning*, and questions of *relationship*. Whether the dying person addresses these questions is entirely up to the individual in his or her own freedom. The fact that some persons freely choose to ignore these questions does not vitiate their importance. Even if all persons were freely to choose to ignore these questions, their importance would not be diminished. Regardless of whether individuals confront these questions, such questions always present themselves as the most obvious and important questions for a dying person to address. Regardless of whether that dying person subscribes to any particular system of religious belief, these questions, as I argue in chapter 2, are aptly described as spiritual.

The first questions are about value. The dying person, at least implicitly, asks questions such as the following: Do I, as an embodied person, now dying, have any value here and now as *me* dying? Has my life, as I have lived it until now, had any value? Will there be anything of value about me that persists after I have died?

The second set of questions is about meaning. The dying person asks questions such as these: Does my dying now, as an embodied person, have any meaning here and now? Has my life, as I have lived it until now, had any meaning? Has there been any meaning in what I have suffered? Will there be any meaning in my living and dying that perdures beyond the moment of my death?

The third set of questions is about relationship. The dying person asks questions such as these: Even as my body breaks and folds, can my interpersonal relationships withstand the blows? Am I really loved by anyone at all? Who are the people whom I have loved and cherished? Will I die as part of a family? Can I be reconciled with those I have wronged and with those who have wronged me? Will my relationships persist beyond the grave?

In most discussions of the care of dying persons, these questions have been subsumed under a set of words that have received far too little serious, critical reflection. These words are invoked continually, as if everyone understood clearly what they mean. Yet the meanings of these words and the questions they evoke in discussions about dying persons rarely are clear. Questions of value often are subsumed under the word *dignity*. Questions of meaning often are subsumed under the word *hope*. Questions of relationship often are subsumed under the term *closure*. These words have served, in some respects, as metaphorical rugs under which all the messy questions about meaning, value, and relationship have been swept. One is left with the appearance of a technically correct, electronically controlled, antiseptically spiritual death. "At Acme HMO, we provide what consumers want: high-quality, cost-effective care at the end of life, giving our patients death with dignity and hope, bringing their lives to gentle closure." Very neat.

Even well-meaning persons concerned with improving the care of dying persons have moved too quickly to package these concerns under very broad labels such as "spiritual suffering" and even dared to try to create quantitative scales to measure (and therefore to control) the spiritual experiences of dying persons. I wonder, however, whether such measurement is even possible. I hear the echoes of questions raised long ago by the prophet Isaiah. "Who has held in a measure the dust of the earth, weighed the mountains in scales and the hills in a balance? Who has directed the spirit of the Lord, or has instructed him as his counselor? Whom did he consult to gain knowledge?" (Is. 40). Even the best health care professionals sometimes are far too uncomfortable with the idea of the unfathomable. Hence, out-comes researchers concerned with care at the end of life try to reduce the spiritual to a check box. Even in the desire to serve the spiritual needs of dying patients, medicine is in danger of sterilizing the spirit right out of dying.

In criticizing some recent approaches to improving the spiritual care of dying persons, I do not wish to imply that health care profes-sionals cannot discuss these issues, grapple with them, and do a better job of facilitating the spiritual work of dying persons. It seems obvious to sensitive clinicians who care for dying persons that whenever dying goes awry—as it often does—frequently it is because either the patient or the caregiver has paid insufficient attention to one or more of these questions of meaning, value, and relationship. We can and should do a better job. All I suggest is that empirical science will not give us the answers to these questions. Total quality management will not redress these deficiencies. The truly spiritual is frightfully unmanageable. Spiri-tual concerns are not glibly resolved by questionnaires. One cannot measure the unmeasureable.

Yet everyone has some intuitive sense of the nature of these spiri-tual questions, particularly as they relate to death. People seem natu-rally to shudder at and recoil from the possibility of death without dignity, hope, or reconciliation. They fear that their own end might be undignified. They wonder if there is anything in which they will be able to hope when their own time comes. They fear alienation and abandon-ment in their final days. Yet too many health care professionals remain fearful of discussing these issues in any depth with their colleagues or their patients.

Dignity

In chapter 3 I discuss dignity in a general way. I now focus on the ques-tion of dignity with respect to the care of dying persons.[1] Although the phrase "death with dignity" has become a slogan for many people, the real meaning of this phrase is anything but clear. Consider that the bill that legalized physician-assisted suicide in the state of Oregon was called the "Death with Dignity Act." Yet many people who opposed the legalization of assisted suicide in that state based their opposition on their belief that assisted suicide is always a violation of the dignity of the dying. Thus, parties to discussions about death with dignity appear to mean different things by *dignity*. The key to understanding these apparently conflicting uses of the word *dignity* is to recall the distinction I make in chapter 3 between attributed dignity and intrinsic dignity.

I also suggest a principle to guide this discussion. Moral words must be used consistently and coherently. This principle implies that whatever one says one means by dignity in discussions of death ought to be the same meaning one assigns to the word in *all* spheres of human moral experience. This conclusion seems unassailably true—and therefore a good place to start.

Dignity, at its root, means worth, stature, or value. Whatever has dignity has value. As I discuss in chapter 3, in the Middle Ages—when the idea of the "Great Chain of Being" dominated metaphysics and cosmology—this concept was very simple. Everything had value, as created by God, and one's value was relative to one's place in the hierarchy of beings. More recently, however, our notion of human dignity has taken a much more egalitarian turn. Although most of us would accept as true that a human being has more value than an ameba, few of us would—and none of us should—accept the notion that a rich person has more dignity than a poor person or that a politician has more dignity than an unelected citizen does. Dignity seems to be something we now attribute to all persons equally, regardless of their station in life. This notion is what I call *intrinsic* dignity—the value one has simply because one is human.

Recall my discussion of Martin Luther King Jr.'s view of intrinsic dignity. He said that he learned this lesson from his grandmother, who told him, "Martin, don't let anyone ever tell you that you're not a somebody."[2] "Somebodiness" captures the core of this notion of intrinsic human dignity. Everybody is a somebody. Even if one rejects the notion of a God before whom all persons are of equal worth, all persons are at least of equal worth before the law.

The relevance of this conception of intrinsic dignity to the care of dying persons should be obvious: Everyone ought to believe that dying persons have no less intrinsic dignity than those who survive them. At least, one ought to believe this if one wishes to be consistent in one's use of moral terms. If this is what intrinsic dignity means in civil rights, this is what it must mean in care at the end of life. That is why beginning this discussion with a principle of consistency is important.

Confusion seems to creep in, however, when people begin to talk about dignity in relation to death. This confusion can be explained if one takes note of the distinction I make in chapter 3 between *attributed* dignity and *intrinsic* dignity. To review, intrinsic dignity is the value people have simply because they are members of the human family. It is the dignity that is *intrinsic* to being human. Attributed dignity, on the other hand, is the value or worth one attributes to others or to oneself. Attributed dignity is based on one's power, one's prestige, one's function, one's productivity, and one's degree of control over one's situation. This sort of dignity depends on how others see us and how we see ourselves. The signs of attributed dignity vary from culture to culture and change over time.

The crux of the matter is this: Terminal illness and death mount a relentless attack on *attributed* dignity. Dying persons look different. They lose their independence. People tell them when they can eat, when they can defecate, and when they can go to sleep. They can't go out to the corner store for coffee and a newspaper. They lose their jobs. People avoid them. Dying brings these changes upon them. The spiritual question about death and dignity, however, is whether such an assault ultimately is complete or whether there is, after all, an intrinsic human dignity that persists even in death.

Donald Hall—husband of the late Jane Kenyon, an American poet who died of leukemia at the end of the twentieth century—is himself a poet. He has written powerful poetry about his wife's death. His words capture the transcendent splendor of the mundane details of dying. The following is an excerpt from his poem "Last Days."

> Incontinent three nights
> before she died, Jane needed lifting
>   onto the commode.
> He wiped her and helped her back into bed.
>   At five he fed the dog
> And returned to find her across the room,
>   Sitting in a straight chair.
> When she couldn't stand, how could she walk?
>   He feared she would fall
> And called for an ambulance to the hospital,
>   But when he told Jane,
> Her mouth twisted down and tears started.
>   "Do we have to?" He cancelled.
> Jane said, "Perkins, be with me when I die."[3]

This poem is about dignity in death. It is about *intrinsic* human dignity persisting in the midst of assaults on attributed dignity. How can a human being appear to walk even when that person is rendered physically incapable of standing? It is through the power of intrinsic dignity. Regardless of whether it is literally true, it is always metaphorically true that the lame can walk in dignity.

Thus, this poem is a proclamation of the intrinsic sense of human dignity that is not lost when a person becomes powerless and dependent. It proclaims the dignity that is not lost as a person becomes disfigured. It proclaims the dignity that does not depend upon how others view us or even how we view ourselves. It is about the dignity that all persons have—the dying no less than the surviving. This dignity is ineradicable. It does not admit of degrees. It does not depend upon how productive one is. It does not depend upon any function one might serve. It is the dignity all human beings have, simply because they are human.

Nor is it up to any individual to decide what constitutes the intrinsic value of any human being, including the individual himself or herself. As Simone Weil observes, perhaps shockingly, the basis of our dignity is not what is most personal and unique about us but what is most impersonal and common: "What is sacred in a human being is the impersonal in him."[4] What seems most trivially true about us—that we are all human beings—grounds our dignity. This concept may come as a shock to Americans. Americans are so caught up in individualism and the language of rights that they may have trouble grasping that the grounds for respecting individual freedom are what is least individual in people.

Dying mounts an assault on the dignity of each dying human being. No one can claim a right not to die. Ineluctably, dying raises questions about one's worth and value as one is dying, about the value of the life one has led up to the moment of death, and about whether anything that is valuable about oneself perdures beyond the moment of death. One's spiritual task as life draws to a close is to reject, discover, recover, or affirm one's own grasp of one's own intrinsic human dignity. As the grounds for *attributed* dignity fade (as they inevitably will for each of us), the question becomes, is that all there is? Is there nothing more about me that is of value except how I feel, how I appear to others, how much I can do without anyone else's help, and how productive I can be? This inquiry may lead to further questions: If there is intrinsic value to my life, what is the source of that value? Can such a belief be validated? Does such value perdure? These questions are spiritual, whether they are raised in a religious context or not. One is free to choose not to grapple with these questions, but they are *obvious*. One also can choose to answer in the negative—to conclude that there is no intrinsic value to human life. To do so, however, one must be consistent in one's belief about the valuelessness of all human life. One should bear in mind that such a response requires no less faith than belief in a divinity that creates, redeems, and sanctifies human life.

Hope

The word *hope*, like the word *dignity*, has been haplessly muddled in discussions about dying. In fact, this muddling probably has been occurring for centuries. The Hippocratic texts, for instance, talk of lying to patients about their diagnoses, so they do not lose hope.[5] Writing in this tradition, Thomas Percival advised, "A physician should not be forward to make gloomy prognostications. . . . For the physician should be the minister of hope and comfort to the sick; that by such cordials to the drooping spirit, he may smooth the bed of death, revive expiring life, and counteract the depressing influences of those maladies which rob the philosopher of fortitude, and the Christian of consolation."[6]

Those of us who care for patients often speak in such ways. We whisper in dark corridors about "hopeless cases." Even with the best of intentions, we write about providing better care for persons who are "hopelessly ill." Families sometimes hesitate to authorize discontinuation of treatment because doing so would signal that they had given up hope.

Is anyone's dying necessarily truly hopeless, however? Do dying persons have anything for which to hope? I think they do, and I urge health care professionals to clean up their language and avoid glibly declaring any patient hopeless.

Naturally, a dying person might *desire* not to die. Most of us who survive them have this same natural desire. No one, however, can really *hope* never to die. All persons are mortal. Therefore, properly speaking, one cannot hope not to die.

One might say of persons who have exhausted all means of cure that their cases are "hopeless." This assessment would be true, however, only if there were nothing more for a human being to desire than long life and the death of tumor cells, HIV virions, and tubercle bacilli. Most persons recognize that human desire is far deeper. At the limit, hope based on needles and pills dissolves into delusion. A proper object of hope must be attainable. Therefore, if one is dying, one's hopes must be deeper than death.

Death is the ultimate human limit. It cannot be avoided. It cannot be wished away. It cannot be prayed away. This was the message Christians believe the Father delivered to Jesus in the Garden of Gethsemane (Luke 22:42). This cup will not pass from any of us.

Ultimate hope, then, is not about a cure for cancer or AIDS. These goals certainly are good things to wish for, but they cannot be the source of ultimate hope. The object of ultimate hope must be located beyond the limits of our finite, corporal, individual existence.

Meaning is such a transcendent object. The object of ultimate hope must be a source of meaning, however one construes it. For Christians, Muslims, and Jews, this transcendent object of desire is the one, holy, all-loving, and almighty God. For persons of other faiths, or of no faith, this object of ultimate, genuine hope must be whatever source of meaning one holds to be prior to or transcend the limits of finite, corporal, individual existence. Vaclav Havel has put it this way: "Hope is definitely not the same thing as optimism. It is not the conviction that something will turn out well, but the certainty that something makes sense, no matter how it turns out."[7]

Rejecting, discovering, recovering, or holding onto an ongoing source of transcendent meaning is one of the major spiritual tasks of dying persons. The opposite of hope is called despair, but despair really is just another name for meaninglessness. Suffering without any sense of meaning is abject hopelessness.

Jane Kenyon, whose husband wrote so movingly about the dignity of her dying, herself wrote eloquently about the hope that can be found in dying. Her poem—written years before her own fatal illness—is called "Let Evening Come."

> Let the light of late afternoon
> shine through chinks in the barn, moving
> up the bales as the sun moves down.
>
> Let the cricket take up chafing
> as a woman takes up her needles
> and her yarn. Let evening come.
>
> Let dew collect on the hoe abandoned
> in long grass. Let the stars appear
> and the moon disclose her silver horn.
>
> Let the fox go back to its sandy den.
> Let the wind die down. Let the shed
> go black inside. Let evening come.

To the bottle in the ditch, to the scoop
in the oats, to air in the lung
let evening come.

Let it come, as it will, and don't
be afraid. God does not leave us
comfortless, so let evening come.[8]

Hope for dying persons lies beyond the limits of what is measurable in the space and time we are allotted on this earth. Beyond the physical realities of suffering and death, either there is meaning or there is not. Evening will come. Whether there is any meaning beyond the horizon of human finitude is an issue each dying person must face.

Reconciliation

When one hears talk of patients' need for closure at the end of life, one should pay close attention. Most often this talk of closure is a way of describing *reconciliation* without having to sound spiritual. The dying person's need for closure is not just about bank accounts but about the need to draw together the raw and painful edges of the wounds that separate people from each other. In our era, contrite recognition of one's faults or admission of one's sense of alienation have come to be regarded as psychopathologies to be overcome or signs of weakness that the prudent person ought never admit. Doctors, nurses, psychologists, social workers, and patients all know that the real need of dying patients is for genuine reconciliation, but they all too often conspire never to speak directly dangerous words such as reconciliation, forgiveness, or love.

What does reconciliation mean? It means restoration of right relationships—with other people, with one's environment, and with one's God. Perhaps the deepest fear of patients with terminal illnesses is that they will be abandoned. Pain hurts. Dying alone, however, amplifies pain beyond what any human being was ever meant to bear.

Human beings' greatest desire is for unconditional love. Each human being knows, however, that his or her own love is always—even at its best—imperfect, conditional, and less than absolute. How can anyone expect anything more from another human being?

The answer, of course, is that one cannot. Sometimes one must come to terms with death to understand this reality. The finitude of our love and the imperfections of our humanity require acknowledgment and forgiveness. One must recognize and forgive the imperfections of family, friends, co-workers, bosses, church, and community. One must recognize one's own imperfect love for all these brothers and sisters and ask for their forgiveness. This is reconciliation. It is an instance of the restoration of right relationship—understanding and acceptance of one's own imperfection.

At the limit, however, this process of reconciliation requires a transcendent term. What if others do not forgive us? What if, in our hardness of heart, our own reconciliation with those who have hurt us is less than pure? Ultimately, the powerful drive within us to be loved is met only if we have faith that there is One who will love and forgive us unconditionally, absolutely, and eternally. Only such love can save us. The dying person must come to grips with the question of whether such love and reconciliation really exist. To die in such love is to die in absolute reconciliation with the universe. To die without it is hell.

John Donne expresses well these needs, questions, and fears in "A Hymn to God the Father," which he is thought to have written in the throes of an illness that almost took his life in 1623.

> Wilt Thou forgive that sin where I begun,
> Which is my sin, though it were done before?
> Wilt Thou forgive those sins through which I run,
> And do them still, though still I do deplore?
> When Thou hast done, Thou hast not done,
> For I have more.
>
> Wilt Thou forgive that sin by which I have won
> Others to sin? And made my sin their door?

> Wilt Thou forgive that sin which I did shun
>> A year or two, but wallowed in a score?
>>> When Thou hast done, Thou hast not done,
>>>> For I have more.
>
> I have a sin of fear, that when I have spun
>> My last thread, I shall perish on the shore;
> Swear by Thyself that at my death Thy Sun
>> Shall shine as it shines now, and heretofore;
>>> And, having done that, Thou hast done.
>>>> I have no more.[9]

In this poem, the speaker struggles with weighty issues such as original sin ("that sin where I begun"), the common human experience of weakness of the will ("and do them still, though still I do deplore"), and inducement of others to evil ("made my sin their door"). He expresses doubts about the truth of the Christian promise of God's forgiveness ("Wilt Thou forgive that sin which I did shun / A year or two, but wallowed in a score"), and the fear that he might die utterly unreconciled, alienated, and alone ("I shall perish on the shore").

This poem, then, clearly is about the need for reconciliation, made acute in the face of death. Donne also puns continuously throughout the poem about his own name and the maiden name of his wife (Ann More). Thus, although the speaker's words are addressed only to God, the field of relationship about which he frets is wider. In typical Donne style, the poem ends on an ambiguous note. The speaker prays desperately that, as he faces death, the Sun (namely Jesus, the Son of God) will shine on him for all eternity and not leave him unreconciled and alienated on the shore. The phrase "Thou hast done. I have no more" subtly suggests the absolute self-surrender of a lover. Having no experience of life after death (an experience none of us have), however, he also fears that such eternal salvation might not really be the absolute universal reconciliation for which he would hope. Perhaps, the poem suggests, God is a jealous lover. The speaker seems to pray for the strength to give himself over completely to God. Yet he also fears that death might bring an eternal life with God alone—an eternal life without his beloved wife. We might read "Thou hast done. / I have no more" as, "You will have John Donne. And John Donne will have no Ann More."

Such hopes and fears express the deep spiritual needs of dying persons for reconciliation, whether they express these needs in such frankly religious language or not. Spirituality is about one's relationship with the transcendent. The relationships on both sides of the horizon of life are caught up in the spiritual. This horizon is always present. Sometimes, however, we just fail to notice it until dusk.

Spirituality and the Care of Dying Persons

Having discussed what I mean by questions of value (i.e., dignity), questions of meaning (i.e., hope), and questions of relationship (i.e., reconciliation), I have an obligation to discuss what these questions mean for health care professionals caring for dying persons. The fundamental point is this: As the foregoing discussion should make clear, health care professionals do not give their patients dignity; they do not give them hope; they do not give them reconciliation. Dignity, hope, and reconciliation are already present as givens in every situation of death. Value is already there, commanding respect. Meaning is already there, awaiting affirmation. Reconciliation presents itself as the already possible restoration of right relationship abiding in the throes of death.

The task of the health care professional is to show respect and reverence for the dignity all dying persons have simply because they are human; to share their own hope that meaning transcends the dying process; and to point the way to reconciliation. They can do nothing more. They must do nothing less. Where possible, health care professionals can create an atmosphere that is conducive to the patient's own grasping of the dignity, hope, and reconciliation that are already there to be grasped. Doctors and nurses should neither be so naïve nor so arrogant as to think that dignity, hope, or reconciliation are theirs to give. Health care professionals who think they are responsible for providing their patients with dignity, hope, and reconciliation will burn out quickly. If they take upon themselves the tasks of offering dignity, hope, and reconciliation, they are doomed to failure—Sisyphus *redux*.

Respecting the intrinsic dignity of dying patients, however, does entail certain concrete moral responsibilities. Respect is not static but dynamic. The link between intrinsic and attributed dignity is forged in moral action. Respect for intrinsic human dignity demands action to build up (to the extent possible) the attributed dignity of human beings—provided this action does not undermine or contradict the intrinsic human dignity that is the ground of moral action. In other words, respect for someone's intrinsic human dignity demands that one show that respect in concrete ways. Saying that one respects the intrinsic dignity of dying persons requires that one assist them in their concrete needs. One shows respect for dying persons by bathing them, feeding them, treating their pain, relieving their nausea, and helping them get out of bed. One shows respect for dying persons by being with them and listening to them attentively, paying careful attention to what they can teach those who survive them.

More than this, however, respect for dying persons requires attention to their spiritual struggles. Health care professionals can point out, by word and action, the dignity that is already there to be grasped by the dying person. Dying persons need to be reminded of their dignity at a time of fierce doubt. They need to understand that they are not grotesque or bothersome; unvalued because they are unproductive; unworthy of time, attention, and resources. Physicians, nurses, and others can help them grasp their own intrinsic dignity with concrete actions that thwart or mitigate the assault that the dying process mounts against their patients' attributed dignity.

Health care professionals also need to create an atmosphere in which dying persons can search for meaning. They need to be open to discussions of spiritual issues and ready to refer their patients to experts in pastoral care who, as part of the team, can assist patients in their struggles with these issues. They can help dying persons by pointing out, through their words and actions, that they themselves do not consider the state of the patient to be hopeless. Instead, they must somehow communicate to dying patients gratitude for the meaning and hope that dying persons freely give to those who care for them. Dying persons can teach nurses, physicians, and other health care professionals countless lessons about life and its meaning every day. These practitioners have only to open their ears and their hearts.

Ultimately, hope is about meaning. Health care professionals can cultivate a spirit of genuine hope in their dying patients only if they themselves lead lives that are anchored by an abiding sense of meaning. That sense of meaning enables them even to heal the dying.

Finally, health care professionals can help patients understand their need for reconciliation. They can break the conspiracy of silence. A physician or nurse can ask a dying patient whether he has told his wife and children, "I love you." Physicians, nurses, and other health care professionals also must understand how much their own relationships with patients can mean to those patients and how important it is to live professional lives that are worthy of the trust that patients have placed in them. Communicating to dying patients that they remain important members of the human community, even as the bonds that keep them and us together are slowly dissolving, is a powerful act of healing. It points the way to the possibility of transcendent love.

Morality, Spirituality, and End-of-Life Care

As important as these spiritual issues might be, one certainly ought never coerce a patient into addressing them. Respect demands that patients be allowed the freedom to choose to ignore these issues or even to answer the ultimate questions in the negative. Although this approach is the right thing to do, giving someone the freedom to die in the belief that life has no intrinsic value, the universe is absurd, and there are no right relationships can be very painful. Caring for such patients can be particularly difficult for persons of faith. Yet one can still believe in that dying patient's dignity; hold out hope for that patient; and remain steadfast in the belief that a compassionate, loving, patient-professional relationship has a transcendent term, even if the patient never acknowledges that any of this might be true. A believer must remember that the freedom not to believe is exactly the freedom that God gives everyone. One should not usurp prerogatives that God has freely abdicated out of his love and respect for the persons he has created.

The dying person brings his or her entire life to the moment of death. Christian theology teaches that if a life has the love of the Incarnate God as the foundation of its value, the source of its hope, and its model of right relationship, this trinity of value, hope, and right relationship is exactly what will be irrevocably, absolutely, and eternally determined in the dying of that person. Caring for a patient who is dying in such a manner is a remarkable privilege. When I enter the room of such a patient (which happens far more often than those who do not care for dying persons might think), I sometimes wonder if I should remove my shoes because I know that the ground on which I am about to tread is holy. I find that I am the one transformed, the one to whom enormous grace has been revealed. Such an experience is more than enough to sustain a doctor or nurse in hospice or palliative care. It is grace enough for the dying.

So let evening come.

Notes

1. Daniel P. Sulmasy, "Death and Human Dignity," *Linacre Quarterly* 61 (Winter (1994)): 27–36.

2. Garth Baker-Fletcher, *Somebodyness: Martin Luther King, Jr. and the Theory of Dignity*, Harvard Dissertations in Divinity, no. 31 (Minneapolis: Fortress Press, 1993), 23.

3. Donald Hall, "Last Days," in *Without* (Boston: Houghton Mifflin, 1998), 41.

4. Simone Weil, "Human Personality," in *The Simone Weil Reader,* ed. G. A. Panichas (New York: David McKay, 1977), 313–39.

5. Hippocrates, Decorum, XVI, in *Hippocrates*, vol. 2, trans. W. H. S. Jones (Cambridge, Mass.: Harvard University Press, 1923), 296–99.

6. Thomas Percival, *Percival's Medical Ethics,* ed. C. D. Leake (Huntington, N.Y.: Robert E. Krieger, 1975), 91.

7. Vaclav Havel, *Disturbing the Peace* (New York: Vintage, 1991), 181.

8. Jane Kenyon, "Let Evening Come," in *Otherwise: New and Selected Poems* (St. Paul, Minn.: Graywolf Press, 1997), 176.

9. John Donne, "A Hymn to God the Father," in *John Donne's Poetry*, ed. A. L. Clements (New York: W. W. Norton, 1966), 94–95.

13

At W;t's End

Efforts among health care professionals to improve the care of dying persons increasingly have begun to include attention to spirituality. This development is wonderful. Hospice workers have instinctually been taking this approach for a long time. With the advent of the new specialty of palliative medicine, academic physicians at teaching hospitals also are beginning to address spiritual themes in their work. Some of these efforts have included making use of literary works to address what is now popularly called the "existential and spiritual suffering" of dying patients. As much as these efforts deserve applause, however, a good deal of this attention misses the mark. To illustrate the possibilities and pitfalls of this approach, consider the play *W;t*, by Margaret Edson, and the reaction of the medical community to this play.[1]

The plot of this Pulitzer Prize–winning drama concerns a woman who is dying of ovarian cancer in an academic medical center. *W;t* attracted enormous critical acclaim and widespread interest among physicians.[2] It was even reviewed in medical journals—a rare event for a work of literature.[3] Furthermore, it has been used for purposes of medical education aimed at improving the care of dying persons.[4] Yet major themes of the play seem to have received little attention, both in informal discussions with physicians and in these reviews. Certainly, some of these reviews have addressed broader themes such as "care" and "abandonment" and the intricacies of the physician-patient relationship. The tendency, however, has been to focus on this play as a satire about the care of dying persons. Although that certainly is true of this multi-layered, intricately woven work of art, such an emphasis does not give the play its due. In a way, saying that *W;t* is a satire about the care of dying persons is like saying that *Hamlet* is a play about royal succession in Denmark. True enough—but something is rotten if we say no more.

The focal point of the play is its protagonist, Vivian Bearing—PhD, professor of English literature, expert on the Holy Sonnets of John Donne—who is coming to grips with her ovarian cancer, her life, and her death. We follow Professor Bearing from her diagnosis through her treatment, aplasia, and sepsis to her death in the throes of an aborted attempt at cardiopulmonary resuscitation despite an order that she not be resuscitated. The play is peppered with flashbacks to Vivian's childhood and her career in academia. Most of the dialogue takes place between Vivian and several health care professionals in the all-too-familiar setting of the "University Comprehensive Cancer Center." This plot is simply a vehicle, however, for a much richer drama. The story of someone dying under the care of doctors is not necessarily a story that is primarily about doctors.

The message of the play is intended for *all* audiences. Only when doctors learn this message will they learn anything really useful from this play. The doctors portrayed in *W;t* don't seem to appreciate this message, and doctors who see or read the play also may fail to appreciate this message. In the graphic words of the play, such a failure would be another "doctor fuckup" (85). Just as the play ends in a mistake, there is a danger that medicine's professional reaction to the play will be a mistake. Physicians, nurses, and other health care professionals may find themselves, like the house officers at the end of the play, "coding a no-code." The only way the play can teach them how to avoid such a mistake is if they realize that the point of the play has both nothing and everything to do with learning how to avoid mistakes. "Herein lies the paradox. John Donne would revel in it" (47).

Two themes that I discuss in details in chapter 12—reconciliation and dignity—are critically important themes in *W;t*. Clinicians who wish to learn from the play would do well to understand these themes.

Reconciliation

Reconciliation is a complex concept. Seeking forgiveness implies recognizing one's own failings. Yet reconciliation also implies the human need to be assured that one is accepted and loved, despite one's failings. It implies a resolution to love and accept others despite their failings— especially the failings of others that have resulted in one's having been hurt or otherwise harmed. Mutual forgiveness fosters reconciliation, but reconciliation is broader than forgiveness. Reconciliation involves a more complete state of acceptance—of the failings of others even when they cannot bring themselves to ask for forgiveness; of the trifold finitude of one's own human condition (physical, intellectual, and moral); of the apparent injustice of the world. To the extent that a dying person can be reconciled, that person attains "closure."

Forgiveness, then, is a major part of reconciliation and closure. The theme of forgiveness emerges subtly, but forcefully, as *W;t* unfolds. Simply put, Vivian spends much of her time on stage asking the audience to forgive her. As the play begins, she states that she's "sorry [she] won't be around" when the doctors ask her corpse, "How are you today?" (5) She later apologizes that her request for a "palliative treatment modality" disrupts "the dramatic coherence of [her] play's last scene." (70) Her "last coherent words" are, "I'm sorry." (73).

In the middle of the play—at its very heart—stands the text of *Donne's Holy Sonnet V, "If poysonous mineralls. . . ." Vivian recites the sonnet and then delivers a lecture on its meaning.*

> If poysonous mineralls, and if that tree,
> Whose fruit threw death on else immortall us,
> If lecherous goats, if serpents envious
> Cannot be damn'd; Alas; why should I bee?
> Why should intent or reason, borne in mee,
> Make sinnes, else equall, in mee, more heinous?
> And mercy being easie, and glorious
> To God, in his sterne wrath, why threatens hee?
> But who am I, that dare dispute with thee?

> O God Oh! of thine onely worthy blood,
> And my teares, make a heavenly Lethean flood,
> And drowne in it my sinnes blacke memorie.
> That thou remember them, some claime as debt,
> I thinke it mercy if thou wilt forget.

This sonnet is a complex plea for God's mercy and forgiveness, spoken by one whose intellect cannot fully accept the possibility of such forgiveness. In the play's wonderful irony (6), the audience grasps that in Vivian's third-person analysis of the poem, she really is talking about herself. To drive this point home, the stage directions state, "VIVIAN *moves in front of the screen and the projection of the poem is cast directly upon her*" (50). From this position she addresses her "class":

> Doctrine assures us that no sinner is denied *forgiveness*, not even one whose sins are an overweening *intellect* or overwrought *dramatics*. The speaker does not need to *hide* from God's judgment, only to accept God's *forgiveness*. It is very simple. Suspiciously simple.

Vivian teeters on the brink of forthrightly understanding her own need for reconciliation with God, death, and other human beings, but the play leaves open to interpretation the question of whether she ever fully resolves these issues. She speaks for the audience as much as for herself when she says:

> But it is too late. The poetic encounter is over. We are left to our own consciences. Have we outwitted Donne? Or have we been outwitted? (50).

Vivian really needs forgiveness. She is one whose "sins are an overweening intellect and overwrought dramatics." Yet the conception that forgiveness might even be possible lies just beyond the grasp of her own keen intellect. She has no idea how to ask for it and considers it easier just to disappear.

Relationship

Reconciliation and the recognition of dignity are actualized only in con-text—the context of relationship. The postdoctoral fellow in the play, Dr. Jason Posner, unwittingly describes the way human relationships form the glue that binds both dignity and forgiveness together when he describes the cellular biology of cancer to his patient, Vivian. In this richly layered dialogue, conducted simultaneously at two levels of in-terpretation, one discovers even more of the play's wonderful irony. Both characters describe an intellectual interest in what they do not possess and profess an intellectual affinity for what they are both studi-ously avoiding even as they speak about it. Jason and Vivian both say that what they find "awesome" about cancer cells is the loss of "contact inhibition." Yet both obviously are inhibited by contact with human be-ings. Jason goes on to state, suggestively, that this loss of contact inhibi-tion is what it means for cells to become immortal (56–57). When Vivian is placed in clinical isolation, she states explicitly that cancer (i.e., loss of contact inhibition) has not driven her into isolation. She has been driven into isolation by the treatment she has received at the hands of her doctors (47). Vivian and her oncologist, Dr. Harvey Kele-kian, really are co-conspirators in this treatment. Vivian's treatment plan is about knowledge and toughness, a way of avoiding both life and death (11–12). In short, her treatment, like her life, is a program for maintaining and restoring contact inhibition.

In their own personal isolated alienation and overintellectualiza-tion, the physicians in the play mirror Vivian, even as she mirrors us, the audience. Vivian's real struggle is not against the cancer but against what the postdoctoral fellow, Jason, correctly calls the theme of "Salva-tion Anxiety" in the poetry of John Donne (75–76). Vivian's anxiety concerns precisely the nexus of relationships that might ultimately carry her past death. That is, her struggle "is ultimately about overcom-ing the seemingly insuperable barriers separating life, death, and eter-nal life" that Donne describes in Holy Sonnet V, "Death, be not proud." (14). Vivian's graduate school mentor, Professor E. M. Ashford, tells her in a flashback, "It is *not wit*, Ms. Bearing. It is truth. The paper's not the point. . . . Don't go back to the library. Go out. Enjoy yourself with your friends" (15).

Like Vivian, Jason understands this point only intellectually. We learn that in living his life, Jason has shunned the "fellowship" part of his postdoctoral fellowship—"the part with the human beings" (57)—in favor of a research career. He is in need of constant reminders to be "clinical" (i.e., human) in his dealings with patients. Dr. Kelekian, the professor of oncology, treats Vivian exactly the way she treats the students in her classes. His patients and her students become pretexts for the display of personal prowess and control—an exercise in wit. Like her doctors, Vivian fears both love and death. Like her doctors, she overintellectualizes all relationships and thereby avoids any need for reconciliation. She never shows any mercy to her students, not even allowing extensions for late term papers—even when the excuse is a death in the family, which she dismisses sarcastically: "Don't tell me. Your grandmother died" (63).

We also learn, slowly, how isolated Vivian's life really is. There are hints of a tough childhood. There is no mention of her mother, other than death. We learn that Vivian preferred the library to the company of her fellow students in graduate school. She is childless and unmarried. Her parents are now dead. Her colleagues fear her. No one visits her in the hospital.

Vivian's relationship with Kelekian also is purely intellectual. We learn that they both decry the dullness of their students (10). To Vivian's delight, after a student answers a question incorrectly during rounds, Dr. Kelekian remarks, "Why do we waste our time, Dr. Bearing?" (39). They exchange knowing winks. Wit keeps people at bay.

At one point in the play Vivian tries to reach out to Jason at a human level, asking him if he ever misses any of his patients. He almost opens up but then quickly turns the conversation into a mental status exam (57–59). Vivian also tries to reach out to the nurse, Susie, who offers Vivian the only meaningful interaction she has with the medical staff anywhere in the play—they share a popsicle together (65–66). Yet Susie also quickly escapes from any deeper interpersonal engagement and turns the conversation into an abstract discussion of the risks and benefits of a "do not resuscitate" (DNR) order (67–69).

Only in the haze of morphine does Vivian manage any interpersonal reconciliation. The painful flashback of her interaction with her father at age five becomes redeemed in her dying days. As the morphine is injected, Vivian shares a joke with Susie about its "soporific" qualities—using the same word that she claims, in her flashback, launched her career. In place of her father, in place of her mother, she receives a visit from her old mentor. Professor Ashford crawls into bed with her and reads for her—not Donne but a children's bunny story like the one in which Vivian, at age five, first read the word "soporific." The scene is quite tender and compassionate. The bunny story and Ashford's own actions are filled with the hope of an unconditional, reconciling love. This is the love and forgiveness that Vivian has always wanted but has never allowed herself to accept.

Dignity

As I have explained, dignity means value or worth. In its *intrinsic* sense, it means the value that each human being has simply because each is human. Although Vivian Bearing does not set out consciously in this direction, her pilgrimage through the play is toward this deeper sense of dignity in the face of the "countless indignities" she suffers (41). She begins by mistaking her intrinsic dignity for her attributed dignity, but gradually, painfully, she learns to tell the difference. She might have thought that her dignity came with the pomp of her title, but her title subtly migrates through the drama from "Doctor" to "Ms." to "Vivian." She might have thought that her dignity was based on her appearance, but she quickly loses her beauty with her publicly vanishing hair (40). She might have thought that her dignity consisted in freedom from pain and enjoyment of life's pleasures, but she loses it in the pain that "hurts like hell" (70) and in the ugly vomitus at the bottom of her plastic washbasin (32). Finally, she learns that her dignity cannot be associated with power and control (48) because her power and control are absent from the play's first moment, tethered to the IV pole she drags with her throughout the play like a ball and chain. In the end, Vivian has to learn that she has no worth or value except herself. The one who recognizes her intrinsic dignity is her true mentor, E. M. Ashford, whose reconciling love is expressed in a kiss: "May flights of angels sing thee to thy rest" (80).

How much of this Vivian understands through the haze of morphine initially is unclear. As the stage directions state, however, just as the play ends—in the throes of her final indignity, in the calamity of the "code on the no-code," in the playing out of an egregious medical mistake—she is described as "naked and beautiful, reaching towards the light" (85).

Lessons for Clinicians

These themes, then, are among the central messages of W;t. At its deepest level, the play is not about health care professionals or the care of dying persons. It is about "Salvation Anxiety"—the question of whether we, as human beings, finally have any worth or value independent of how we appear to others or what we think of ourselves; whether we can recognize this value in each other; whether we can reconcile ourselves to each other for our individual and collective failures to treat each other with such dignity; whether we can allow ourselves, finally, to be loved and forgiven; and whether this reconciliation ultimately saves us in any way. Like Vivian, all of us one day will take our final exam. Like Vivian, however, we don't understand the question—and time is running out (70).

To seek forgiveness, we must first understand that we have done wrong. This acknowledgment is where physicians and other health care professionals can benefit most from this play. We need to learn, at least as professionals, what is broken in our relationships. We need to learn what we must say (coherently) that we are sorry for. We do not learn from W;t any useful lines we can use with patients, nor should we be led to believe that we can even learn which turns of phrase are especially unhelpful. It is not *W;t*. It is truth. The play is not the point. What we need to learn is that we must be persons of reconciling love before we will ever be equipped to meet the needs of dying persons. That is a tall order.

Beyond W;*t*'s End

For what do we, as health care professionals—particularly physicians—need forgiveness? The play does not tell us everything, but it invites us, as persons, to ask this question. Collectively, as a profession of persons, we can begin to ask this question of ourselves. Grappling with this question may help make us better healers.

We need forgiveness, first, for our failure to recognize the intrinsic dignity of our patients as persons.[5] For the times we have treated them merely as objects of science or profit.[6] For the times we have failed to learn from them as persons—learning only, as Vivian Bearing accuses Dr. Kelekian, enough to write papers about their ovaries (53). For our insensitivity, when we have acted like Jason—who does a pelvic examination, notes a problem, is unable to conceal his surprise at the findings, and never mentions it again to his terrified patient (31). For the times we have kept our patients at bay, overintellectualized our clinical world, and created an atmosphere of isolation for them and for ourselves.[7] For the times we have lied to our patients—"You're doing swell. Isolation is no problem. Couple of days. Think of it as a vacation" (46).

We need forgiveness, second, from each other. For our petty jealousies, backbiting, and detracting ("subservience, hierarchy, gratuitous displays, sublimated rivalries"; 37). For our cutthroat competitiveness as students, as well as in our practice and academic settings.[8] For our overly harsh educational system, which teaches by humiliation and sleep deprivation—"Wake me up when the counts come back from the lab" (45).[9] For our collective denial of death and our failure to realize the limitations of our craft.[10]

Finally, we need to forgive ourselves or allow ourselves to be forgiven.[11] For our individual limitations as practitioners. For the patients we've harmed through our ignorance, our rashness, or our indecisiveness, whether culpable or not.[12] For our failure to embrace our own humanity, with its intrinsic dignity and its limitations, casting ourselves in the roles of the superheroes we are not.[13] Our most profound dignity comes not from our roles as health care professionals but from the fact that we are persons.[14]

Unless we are prepared to deal with these issues of dignity and reconciliation in our own lives, we will not be able to deal with them in the lives of the persons we serve. We share Vivian Bearing's predicament: "I thought being extremely smart would take care of it. But I see that I have been found out" (70).

Is what comes between life and death a mere comma's worth of breath, or is the gap as wide as a semicolon (15)? Like John Donne, like Vivian Bearing, like Harvey Kelekian, we all face this question, each in our own way. We each answer in our own way. Like our patients, we have heard of "this promise of salvation," and like them we "just can't deal with it" (76).

This promise has been written in the sometimes disappearing ink of dignity and forgiveness. Hence, with fierce doubts, we face the play's starkly contradictory conclusion: "It [the promise of salvation] just doesn't stand up to scrutiny. But you can't face life without it either" (76). Dying persons, especially, are painfully aware of this paradox. Until we realize that it is our paradox as well, however, Margaret Edson's brilliant play will be lost on us. We will go on playing our usual roles as just the sorts of persons about whom satires will be written. If so, let us hope that our patients forgive us anyway.

Notes

1. Margaret Edson, *W;t* (New York: Faber and Faber, 1999). Parenthetical references in the text of this chapter are to page numbers in this edition of the play.

2. Abigail Zuger, "A Turn for the Worse in the Image of Physicians," *New York Times* (December 15, 1998), D4.

3. Faith McLellan, "Medical Writings: *W;t*," *Annals of Internal Medicine* 131 (1999): 718–19; Abraham Philip, "*W;t*: A Play," *Journal of the American Medical Association* 283 (2000): 3261.

4. M. J. Friedrich, "*W;t*: A Play Raises Issues of Emotional Needs of Patients," *Journal of the American Medical Association* 282 (1999): 1611–12.

5. Paul Ramsey, *The Patient as Person* (New Haven, Conn.: Yale University Press, 1970).

6. Charles J. Dougherty, "The Costs of Commercial Medicine," *Theoretical Medicine* 11 (1990): 275–86.

7. Anthony L. Suchman and Dale A. Matthews, "What Makes the Patient-Doctor Experience Therapeutic? Exploring the Connexional Dimension of Medical Care," *Annals of Internal Medicine* 108 (1988): 125–30.

8. Robert Coles, "The Moral Education of Medical Students," *Academic Medicine* 73 (1998): 55–57; Victoria Akre, Erik Falkum, Bjørn Hofvedt, and Olaf G. Aasland, "The Communication Atmosphere between Physician Colleagues: Competitive Perfectionism or Supportive Dialogue?" *Social Science and Medicine* 44 (1997): 519–26; Joanna Jones-Ellis and Donald R. Inbody, "Psychotherapy with Physicians' Families: When Attributes in Medical Practice Become Liabilities in Family Life," *American Journal of Psychotherapy* 42 (1988): 380–83.

9. Dimitri A. Christakis and Chris Feudtner, "Ethics in a Short White Coat: The Ethical Dilemmas that Medical Students Confront," *Academic Medicine* 68 (1993): 249–54; Donald G. Kassebaum and Ellen R. Cutler, "On the Culture of Student Abuse in Medical School," *Academic Medicine* 73 (1998): 1149–58; Gary S. Richardson, James K. Wyatt, Jason P. Sullivan, E. John Orav, Allan E. Ward, Marshall A. Wolf, and Charles A. Czeisler, "Objective Assessment of Sleep and Alertness in Medical House Staff and the Impact of Protected Time for Sleep," *Sleep* 19 (1996): 718–26.

10. Christopher Meyers, "The Impact of Physician Denial upon Patient Autonomy and Well-Being," *Journal of Medical Ethics* 18 (1992): 135–37; Daniel Callahan, "Death and the Research Imperative," *New England Journal of Medicine* 342 (2000): 654–56.

11. Lane A. Gerber, "A Piece of My Mind: Forgiveness," *Journal of the American Medical Association* 259 (1988): 2461.

12. Michael A. LaCombe, "Seeking Forgiveness," *Annals of Internal Medicine* 130 (1999): 444–45; Albert W. Wu, Thomas A. Cavanaugh, Stephen J. McPhee, Bernard Lo, and Guy P. Micco, "To Tell the Truth: Ethical and Practical Issues in Disclosing Medical Mistakes to Patients," *Journal of General Internal Medicine* 12 (1997): 770–75; John F. Christensen, Wendy Levinson, and Patrick M. Dunn, "The Heart of Darkness: The Impact of Perceived Mistakes on Physicians," *Journal of General Internal Medicine* 7 (1992): 424–31.

13. Richard L. Mabry, "The Physician and the Jehovah Complex," *Southern Medical Journal* 84 (1991): 684.

14. Abraham J. Heschel, "The Patient as a Person," in *The Insecurity of Freedom* (New York: Noonday Press/Farrar, Strauss, and Giroux, 1966), 24–38; Daniel P. Sulmasy, "Is Medicine a Spiritual Practice?" *Academic Medicine* 74 (1999): 1002–5.

$\underset{\mathclap{\text{\tiny $\sim\!\!\infty$}}}{}$ 14

Peg

It is a philosophical truism that all people are mortal. This premise is not difficult to grasp cognitively. For those of us who are clinicians, it means that all of our patients are going to die, and some will die prematurely. Too often, we speak and act as if this fact were something other than the surest thing we know in medicine. Collective denial can go only so far, however. As pediatric oncologist David Freyer notes, "Although more [patients] are surviving cancer than ever before, decades of progress have not lessened the frustration and sorrow we too experience when our patients die, as many still do."[1]

We know that physicians in the United States have been slow learners with regard to death and dying. The hospice movement in this country developed because physicians paid no attention to the real needs of dying patients, and nurses and community volunteers took matters into their own hands. Better late than never, physicians now are joining the club, as witnessed by the incipient palliative care movement in this country. Bereavement seems to be a new frontier. Although there are no good data, most commentators suggest that U.S. physicians have trouble thinking that they have medical responsibilities toward the persons left behind by patients who die.[2] Serious training and research in caring for bereaved persons is only beginning.

If bereavement care for families and friends of deceased patients is a new frontier, however, health professionals' own sense of loss must be somewhere on another planet. There is almost no empirical literature on this topic other than one recent qualitative study from the United Kingdom.³ The results of this study are not surprising. Many physicians reported feeling guilt about their patients who died—fears of having missed something, of not having done enough, or even of having made a mistake. Oddly, physicians in this study reported making contact with bereaved loved ones after the patient's death more often in cases of sudden death than in the setting of long-standing patient-physician relationships. Some study respondents spoke spontaneously of their sense of loss when their patients died.

Psychiatrist Jimmie Holland has speculated about why physicians are so reluctant to reach out to the bereaved loved ones of their deceased patients.⁴ Her speculations help to amplify and interpret the British empirical study. In asking why physicians have been reluctant to attend to the needs of bereaved persons, Holland recounts cases in which physicians have felt guilty when their patients have died, expressed in phrases such as, "I should have done more." She notes that some physicians fear becoming too tied up in bereaved families' emotional maelstroms and therefore hesitate to contact them. Some physicians have been forthcoming about their feelings of loss and how they have become paralyzed by these feelings. Finally, Holland notes the ubiquitous use of the "I'm too busy" excuse to cover up all of these significant emotions.

Boyle has described this cover-up phenomenon as "pulling the curtain closed."⁵ He describes a very familiar scene in a suggestive, literary style. He notes the way in which efforts at resuscitation are conducted—with a mixture of science, command and control, and dark humor, all taking place behind a curtain while the family waits outside, anxious, upset, and sobbing. One by one, as the unsuccessful attempt at resuscitation comes to an end, the residents part the curtain, peek outside, wipe the smiles from their faces, and put on a somber and serious look as they file silently past the family. We all tend to "pull the curtain closed." We deal with loss by putting it at bay—grimness wrapped in a shroud of silence, scientific banter, dark humor, and a stiff upper lip—behind the curtain.

W;t Again

This dynamic is at play in the Pulitzer Prize–winning drama W;t, which I describe in detail in chapter 13. I argue that the play's central themes are spiritual—about life, death, and our deep human need for love. The play highlights many of the ways people in the twenty-first century attempt to ignore these questions. This assessment is at least as true of health care professionals as of patients. The following excerpt of a conversation between the patient-protagonist of W;t, Vivian Bearing, and her postdoctoral oncology fellow, Jason Posner, makes this conclusion clear:

> JASON: Me? Oh, I've got a couple of ideas, things I'm kicking around. Wait till I get a lab of my own. If I can survive this . . . *fellowship.*
> VIVIAN: The part with the human beings.
> JASON: Everybody's got to go through it. All the great researchers. They want us to converse intelligently with clinicians. As though the researchers were the impediments. The clinicians are such troglodytes. So swarmy. Like we have to hold hands to discuss creatinine clearance. Just cut the crap, I say.
> VIVIAN: Are you going to be sorry when I—Do you ever miss people?
> JASON: Everybody asks that. Especially girls.
> VIVIAN: What do you tell them?
> JASON: I tell them yes.
> VIVIAN: Are they persuaded?
> JASON: Some.[6]

When our patients die, we fail to note the fact that we too have a deep need to know that we will be missed when we die and that we need to love others enough to miss them. Death has a way of making plain what is really important. As we see this happening for our patients, if any spark of spiritual life still stirs within us, we are automatically reminded of our own vulnerability and our own deepest needs.

Consider what one resident wrote in a medical publication regarding the death of a patient for whom she had cared in the ICU:

Although confident that her death was for the best, my inability to save her left me with a sense of inadequacy. I was permeated by a huge sense of loss—the loss of my patient, the loss of a life.

As I walk[ed] home alone, I [couldn't] stop thinking about Muriel's family. Her husband's creased forehead, the tears in her children's eyes. Do they know how they . . . moved me? Do they know the heartache I feel over their loss? Do they know I am still thinking of Muriel as I walk down the corridor, ride the elevator, and escape the hospital walls? I can still feel my fingers on her skin, searching for her pulse but finding none. Time of death, 5:13 pm.[7]

Peg

In this chapter I share the story of one of my patients who died. This story will be what sociologists and some moral philosophers call a "thick description"—as opposed to the succinct, efficient, crisp, but ultimately "thin" case descriptions to which physicians are accustomed. This thick description holds the necessary data for thinking about spirituality, death, and patient care. The truth is in the details, or at least among them. It is the story of a woman I call Peg.

Peg was a "fascinoma": a thirty-eight-year-old woman with a history of Peutz-Jegher Syndrome—a rare genetic disorder associated with increased pigmentation of the mouth and a predisposition to cancer, especially colon cancer. In April 1997 she was diagnosed with adenoma malignum (an atypical adenocarcinoma of the cervix known to be associated with Puetz-Jegher syndrome).[8] For all of her life Peg had been the model of a patient with a genetic predisposition to cancer and had faithfully participated in all recommended screening tests. Unfortunately, however, Pap smears only screen for squamous cell cancer. By the time she first noted bloating and abdominal discomfort, she had developed a large tumor mass, peritoneal implants, and ascites.

The prognosis for this cancer is grave.[9] Even with pelvic exenteration (i.e., removal of her ovaries, fallopian tubes, uterus, bladder, rectum, and any visible tumor) followed by combination chemotherapy, there are no long-term survivors. The patient, an attorney, learned all this through her own reading and by seeking opinions at three leading academic cancer centers. She was referred to me by a colleague who knew her socially; my colleague stated that Peg was not interested in surgery or chemotherapy but might be interested in alternative treatments, and she could not find a gynecologic oncologist willing to accept her under those circumstances.

Peg was an attractive, thin woman with expressive blue eyes and blonde hair. She reported that the oral mucosal pigmentation associated with her genetic disorder had disappeared after her teenage years. She had never been married. Her mother had died of a Peutz-Jegher–related cancer at a young age. She was completely estranged from her father, who had abused her as a child. She had no brothers or sisters. She said that she belonged to no church group or other equivalent social organization but that her friends had agreed to help her face the disease. She asked penetrating questions and kept notes on a legal pad at every visit. She wanted a physician who would help her sort out her options and provide medical backup as she pursued alternative treatment options. She handed me several articles from medical journals describing her condition. She already understood what was written in the articles. She did not want to have "surgery and chemotherapy that will only make me sick when I'm going to die anyway."

The first day Peg and I met, we agreed that she would not be resuscitated or intubated. I urged her to fill out an advance directive, giving one of her friends durable power of attorney for health care. At that time, acetaminophen with codeine was sufficient to control her symptoms. I agreed to send laboratory data to any alternative treatment program she wished to pursue and help her sort out alternative treatment regimens.

By October 1997 it was clear that the nonstandard immunomodulatory treatment program on which Peg had embarked was not effective (I never thought it would be, but I knew that trying it was important to her). Her tumor was growing and was now easily palpable on abdominal exam. She was losing weight, and I was now treating her pain with fentanyl patches. She needed laxatives to prevent constipation. She had been experiencing a lot of vaginal bleeding and embarrassing, spontaneous, clear mucinous discharges. When her hematocrit dropped to 21 percent, she received a blood transfusion, which boosted her energy. She was soon experiencing frequent bouts of uncontrolled singultus (hiccups). Chlorpromazine seemed to help. She had frequent waves of nausea, and we progressed through a series of anti-emetics, from prochlorperazine to ondansetron. She needed help sleeping, and soon zoldipem was not enough. As her sleep became worse and her pain required four maximum-strength fentanyl patches, we switched to triazolam and long-acting oral morphine. She reacted badly to the combination, however; she reported feeling "not herself." I thought the problem was the triazolam, but she insisted it was the morphine. What can one do with a patient who is a lawyer? I made a plea bargain. We changed both—to flurazepam and methadone.

Peg felt much better for the next month. She was using oxycodone for breakthrough pain, but her pain was mostly controlled with the methadone. I signed the papers she gave me so she could collect her life insurance policy early. She began to ask how much longer she had. I said, "Months, perhaps. It could be longer or it could be sooner. But now, more than ever, it seems best to take each day on its own terms."

Peg's vaginal discharges had ceased weeks before, presumably as the tumor had closed off her cervix. Her nausea became worse, however, and despite initial relief with a concoction of decadron, diphenhydramine, and chlorpromazine taken by rectum (recommended by the hospice nurses), she began to vomit more frequently. She became dehydrated, and we treated her with intravenous fluids over a few hours in our outpatient observation unit. She felt much better and went home.

Inexplicably, Peg's nausea never really returned. At this point, however, she was spending most of the day in bed. Through it all, however, she never lost her alertness or the brightness in her eyes.

Two weeks later, Peg began to complain that her abdomen had become much more swollen and uncomfortable. We performed a therapeutic paracentesis, removing three liters of malignant ascitic fluid.

I asked Peg what the hardest part about being so sick was. She said, "Seeing myself lose so much weight and seeing my face changing." I did not know what to say. Stumbling, I replied, "I can only imagine what you're going through. Your friends love you a great deal, you know. They're with you. And I promise I'll continue to do what I can for you."

"How much longer now?" she asked.

"I think you'll make it through the holidays," I said. "No promises, but I think so."

Peg's friends were amazing. They had come together, along with the hospice nurses, to form a "share the care" group. I inquired about Peg's spiritual needs and assured her that I was praying for her. She had been raised Roman Catholic but had fallen away from the church. I offered her the services of our pastoral care team, but she said she wasn't interested. During one of Peg's outpatient visits, a medical student who was working with me disclosed to Peg that her mother's prayer group was praying for her. Tears welled up in the eyes of both patient and student. Peg could only manage to say to my student, "Thank you. That's sweet." That was more than enough.

Peg received one further large-volume paracentesis a week later—five liters this time. It was enough; the fluid never reaccumulated.

Just after Christmas, Peg spent a few days in the inpatient hospice for a respite for her caregivers and for some moderate delirium (which cleared when we switched back to flurazepam and stopped the lorazepam that a colleague on call one night had prescribed). When Peg's delirium cleared, she said she didn't want to stay in the hospice any longer. I tried to convince her to stay, but she would have none of it. "I want to be in my own bed. I'm in control in my own apartment. It's quieter there." Peg's death was her own. She would live it out in her own way. How could we interfere? We started a subcutaneous morphine infusion and sent her home.

During the following week, Peg grew progressively weaker. Friends visited. With the money from her life insurance policy, she could afford around-the-clock nursing. Peg's friends report that she was only a little confused. "Is this really cancer I have?" she asked one day. "Yes it is, Peg," they answered. "Aha," she said. "Cancer, it seems, poses many interesting challenges."

I made only one home visit—the night Peg died. I reassured her best friend, who was troubled by the fact that she found herself urging the use of increased morphine for Peg. She was worried that she was hastening Peg's death and doing something wrong. I reassured her that what she was doing was perfectly appropriate, even for very conservative moralists, under the "rule of double effect."[10] "The biggest mistake people make is to underdose patients in these situations," I told her. "You're doing the right thing. Don't worry."

Peg was now barely conscious. Even the day before, however, she had been lucid enough to have insisted on using the bedside commode ("When she couldn't stand, how could she walk?"). Even now, at the end, she had raised her eyebrows in recognition when I arrived. "The journey is coming to a close," I said. "You've raced on ahead of us all, but don't forget us. We won't forget you."

Multiple candles burned softly throughout the apartment. The Christmas tree was still up, and the lights were still on, a full week past the Epiphany. I felt Peg's thready pulse and assured her friend that it wouldn't be long. "Stay with her," I said, knowing she already knew to do so.

Four hours later the hospice nurse paged me at home to let me know that Peg had died.

Of course, I went to her funeral. I do not think there was any way I could not have gone. I needed to be there for Peg. I needed to be there for her friends. I needed to be there for me. She was one of those special patients—perhaps because, in a form of transference, she had come to see me as a father figure. Perhaps because she was about my age, I had taken on—in a form of countertransference—aspects of the role of husband. I had become close to her, and I had to mourn her loss. I had to let God know that I had done my best as her physician. Imperfect as I am, as a physician and as a human being, I needed to know that this was enough. Practicing a finite and fallible craft, I serve finite and fallible creatures. I needed to hear the words of the scripture read at her funeral: "For now we see in a mirror, dimly, but then we shall see face to face. Now I know only in part; then I will know fully, even as I have been fully known" (1 Cor. 13:12).

I had to be connected to the reality of Peg's death—to understand it not just as a notation in a chart but viscerally: to see the dirt poured over her grave. I needed to know more completely how things had turned out. For instance, Peg's father was not at the funeral. There had been no magic reconciliation of the sort I had secretly hoped might happen for her. For all the sometimes facile talk in the palliative care world of helping dying patients come to gentle closure, we all really know that closure is never complete. The dead bring all their untied endings with them. Peg was no exception. She had disappointed me by refusing my offers to have her see a chaplain. I had wanted religious reconciliation for her. Much to my surprise, however, I found out at her funeral that she had been talking with a priest all along. I am told that she gladly agreed to be anointed, she took communion, and she seemed to feel at peace. She had been reconciled to the church, and I was glad for her. The priest, Father Mudd, presided at her funeral, and I met him there—a nice man.

Several years had passed since I had thought about Peg before she rushed back into my mind as I was writing this chapter. I had written out many of these details six years ago and shared them with students in my medical school class on spirituality and medicine. In reviewing Peg's story again, however, I was struck that her dying and her death were fairly ordinary. I began to fear that this story was so routine that it might bore readers. Peg was no saint; I was no hero. We merely developed an attachment, as is common for physicians with patients. This story is but one, among thousands like it. Jimmie Holland calls the reactions we have to our dead patients "mini-griefs."[11] Some are less "mini" than others, but they are all griefs. Telling at least some of these stories, however, routine as they might be, is necessary to remind us of who we are as persons practicing medicine and who our patients are as persons. Hence, a routine story like Peg's is perfect for a reflection such as this.

How?

Where does this story leave clinicians in a practical sense? Does this chapter have any "learning objectives"? Several lessons can be gleaned from this material.

First, clinicians need to step out from "behind the curtain" and acknowledge that they do experience a sense of loss when their patients die. This loss is not the deep bereavement that accompanies the loss of family members, but each death is a real loss. Clinicians need to acknowledge that this loss is real—and that it affects them.

Second, reaching out to loved ones after a patient dies can be helpful not only to the loved ones but also to the health care practitioner. Research shows that families appreciate the contact. Moreover, acknowledging the loss also helps clinicians make their own "mini-griefs" more explicit. A call or even a note will do.

Third, one can think about attending patients' funerals. Obviously, clinicians whose patients die frequently, such as oncologists and intensive care unit nurses, cannot do this for every death. Going to funerals would become a part-time job in itself. I don't know whose funerals one should attend. I suspect one should attend the funerals of patients to whom one felt closest or perhaps those one thinks one failed the most. I have no secret formula to offer other health care professionals. I do know that on certain occasions we clinicians need to attend funerals—for ourselves at least as much as for the patients' families and friends.

Fourth, health care professionals can end the conspiracy of silence among themselves and begin to acknowledge their feelings of loss to each other. Some places have even institutionalized this practice. The Pediatric Intensive Care Unit at Boston Children's Hospital, for instance, holds a monthly multidisciplinary session in which staff members talk about one death that occurred in their unit. They share how they felt, what they most remember, what went well and what did not. Memorial Sloan Kettering and the de Vos Cancer Centers hold similar sessions.[12] Such sessions improve the quality of care, although such improvements are not the kind for which we will ever develop measurement instruments.

Finally, as I recommend throughout this book, if one has a spiritual life, religious or not, it pays to cultivate one's own spirit. Health care is hard work. Treating patients and then losing them is intense. The questions of meaning, value, and relationship that arise naturally in the course of treatment, however—for health professionals as well as for patients—are genuine spiritual questions with which to struggle.[13] Some preliminary data even suggest that oncology staff members who cultivate their own spiritual lives are relatively protected against burnout.[14]

Death is inevitable. It is more mysterious than life itself. Understanding how it affects those of us who care for patients who die will make us all better healers.

Notes

1. David R. Fryer, "This Work We Do: Reflections from a Pediatric Hematology/Oncology Memorial Service," *Journal of Pediatric Hematology/Oncology* 23 (2001): 213–14.

2. David Casarett, Jean S. Kutner, Janet Abrahm, and the End-of-Life Care Consensus Panel, "Life after Death: A Practical Approach to Grief and Bereavement," *Annals of Internal Medicine* 134 (2001): 208–15.

3. Eric M. Saunderson and Leone Ribsdale, "General Practitioners' Beliefs and Attitudes about How to Respond to Death and Bereavement: A Qualitative Study," *British Medical Journal* 319 (1999): 293–96.

4. Jimmie C. Holland, "Management of Grief and Loss: Medicine's Obligation and Challenge," *Journal of the American Medical Women's Association* 57 (Spring 2002): 95–96.

5. W. Richard Boyle, "The Curtain: What Happens When Doctors Reach Out to Bereaved Family Members," *Health Affairs* 21 (July–August 2002): 242–45.

6. Margaret Edson, *W;t* (New York: Faber and Faber, 1999), 57–58.

7. Jennifer L. Rosenblum, "Why I Still Cry: Sharing a Young Internist's Reflections on the Death of a Patient at the End of a Long Day," *Medical Economics* 79 (July 2002): 65–66.

8. Preeti J. Srivatsa, Gary L. Keeney, and Karl C. Podratz, "Disseminated Cervical Adenoma Malignum and Bilateral Ovarian Sex Cord Tumors with Annular Tubules Associated with Peutz-Jeghers Syndrome," *Gynecologic Oncology* 53 (1994): 256–64.

9. C. Blake Gilks, Robert H. Young, P. Aguirre, Ronald A. DeLellis, and Robert E. Scully, "Adenoma Malignum (Minimal Deviation Adenocarcinoma) of the Uterine Cervix: A Clinicopathological and Immunohistochemical Analysis of 26 Cases," *American Journal of Surgical Pathology* 13 (1989): 717–29.

10. Daniel P. Sulmasy and Edmund D. Pellegrino, "The Rule of Double-Effect: Clearing Up the Double-Talk," *Archives of Internal Medicine* 159 (1999): 545–50.

11. Holland, "Management of Grief and Loss."

12. Fryer, "This Work We Do"; Holland, "Management of Grief and Loss."

13. Daniel P. Sulmasy, *The Healer's Calling* (New York: Paulist Press, 1997); idem, "Is Medicine a Spiritual Practice?" *Academic Medicine* 74 (1999): 1002–5; idem, "A Biopsychosocial-Spiritual Model for Care at the End of Life," *The Gerontologist* 42 (2002, suppl. 3): 24–33.

14. Kathryn M. Kash, Jimmie C. Holland, William Breitbart, S. Berenson, J. Dougherty, S. Ouellette-Kobasa, and L. M. Lesko, "Stress and Burnout in Oncology," *Oncology* 14 (2000): 1621–37.

Postscript
Is There Life after the Clinic?

This book has been a start. Although much remains to be done, I hope this book has been a beginning.

I am fully aware that much of what I have written here will be controversial, both inside and outside the broad spirituality and medicine "movement." I wrote this book in dialogue, however, with many scholars who have weighed in on recent debates about spirituality and health care. I hope this book stimulates an even deeper and more constructive dialogue among us.

Nonetheless, I wrote this book believing the critics to be a minority. Conversations with my colleagues have led me to believe that many health care professionals are looking for a new future for health care. Medicine can no longer afford to cling to a reductionistic form of practice as applied science, nor can medicine jettison science and replace it with shamanistic revivalism. What we need is a dialectically synthetic future that will reconcile all these concerns into a new and dynamic form of practice. However imperfectly, the path I outline in this book points in that direction.

I believe that growing numbers of practitioners take the transcendent questions of meaning, value, and relationship seriously and are aware of the importance of these questions in the lives of their patients. Religious or not, these practitioners have had their fingers on the pulse of practice and have been the first to recognize that Foucault's clinic is dead. They are searching for something new. If I am correct in naming that search as a spiritual quest, then this book may help point the way to a possible life for these practitioners and their patients after the death of the clinic. In this book I only outline the potential shape of this new form of practice. I point in a few directions, give a few hints, make a few guesses. Much remains to be done, and I certainly will not accomplish all of it. I have suggested a measured course—a way forward toward a biopsychosocial-spiritual form of health care. I am hopeful about the future. I am convinced that the *spirit* of medicine is too powerful to be crushed by any social or historical force. Medicine needs a scientific basis—but it also needs a soul.

Emily Dickinson was right. We must be very careful.

Index

Adinolfi, M., 51
Alameda County study of religious practice and health care outcomes, 164
Alexander the Great, 47
American Medical Association (AMA), 16
Aquinas, Thomas, 27–28, 63
Aristotle, 27
Augustine, St., 195

Ben Sira: the author, 46; and covenantal relationships, 56, 75; and "Deuteronomic retribution," 52–53; and Greek influence on Jewish medicine, 47–48, 49–50, 52, 75; healing and magic, 51; and "honor" due to physicians, 54; and Jewish wisdom literature, 47–48; and legitimacy of medical profession, 51–53; and medicine as dynamic, 53–54; and medicine in Jewish history, 48–51; and Oath of Asaph, 51; and the patient's role/responsibility in healing, 55–56; the physician's duty and right to heal, 51–52; reconciling Jewish tradition and new medical knowledge, 52, 53–54; the text and translation, 45–46; and the "therapeutic moment," 54–55; verse 5 and Exodus, 53–57; the Wisdom of, 44–59

Berlant, Jeffrey Lionel, 98
biopsychosocial-spiritual model of health care, 121–46; alternative biopsychosocial models of the 1970s, 122–23; and bereavement processes, 139; and data on effectiveness of spiritual interventions, 136–37; determining proper roles of all parties, 136; disease in, 125; holistic healing and restoration of right relationships, 126–28; and humanities research, 139; illness in, 125–26; intrinsic spirituality and the human being-in-relationship, 125–26; measurement domains, 130–33; measurement domains, interaction of, 134–35, 136; measuring religiosity, 130–31; measuring spiritual/religious coping and support, 132; measuring the spiritual, 129–30, 132–33; measuring value and meaning (dignity and hope), 135–36; and patients' interest in having clinicians address their spiritual concerns, 128–29; and professionals' spirituality, 138–39; and quality of life, 132–33, 134–35, 139; religion, defining, 124; research agenda and future topics, 135–39, 140; spirituality, defining, 124; and spiritual significance of

biopsychosocial-spiritual model of
health care (*continued*)
patient-professional relationships,
137; and tools for taking spiritual
histories, 137–38
Bolus (Democritus) of Mendes, 50
Bonaventure, St., 65
Boston Children's Hospital, Pediatric
Intensive Care Unit, 233
Bowne, Helen Yoo, 11
Boyle, W. Richard, 225
Byrd, Randolph, and study of inter-
cessory prayer, 147, 152, 153, 154

CAGE questions for alcoholism
screening, 138, 145n55
care, 3–12; cultivating, 8–11; and
Dickinson poem, 3–6, 8–9; for difficult patients, 41–42; as patients'
worries or anxieties, 9; and recognition of the mystery of Life, 5–7,
10–11; as solicitude, 9; as treatment, 9
case presentations, aesthetics of, 4–5
Cassell, Eric, 86n10
Catechism of the Catholic Church,
192, 193–94
Cerullo, Michael A., 151–52, 156
Cheney, Dick, 121
Chibnall, John T., 151–52, 156
Chochinov, Harvey, 135–36
Cicero, 27
Cohen, Cynthia B., 156
collaborative model, 180–81, 182–83
compassion, 65–66, 84
Conley, John, 10
consumerism, medical, 79, 80
Copernicus, Nicolaus, 28
covenants, 56, 75, 82–85

death and dying, spiritual issues of,
187–88, 197–212, 213–23,
224–35; and biopsychosocial-spiritual model of health care, 139;

and creation of atmospheres conducive to dignity, hope, and reconciliation, 209–11; death-with-
dignity discussions, 199–201; dignity issues, 199–203, 210, 219–20;
Edson's *W;t* and themes of dignity
and reconciliation, 213–23, 226;
hope and questions of meaning,
203–6; lessons for health care professionals, 220–21, 232–34; new
bereavement care in American
medicine, 224–25; and paradoxes
of life and death, 6–7; and patients'
funerals, 233; "Peg," 227–32; and
physicians' guilt, 224–27; questions about meaning, 197–98,
203–6, 210–11; questions dying
persons must address, 197–99;
and reaching out to bereaved loved
ones, 225–27, 233; reconciliation
and forgiveness, 215–16, 221–22;
reconciliation and questions of relationship, 206–9, 211; respecting
patients' demands for freedom to
die, 211–12; and spiritual lives of
health care professionals, 233–34
Death Transcendence scale, 133
Declaration of Geneva, 96
de Vos Cancer Center, 233
dialectic of healing and spirituality,
60–88; and beings-in-relationship,
63, 64–65; and compassion,
65–66; and covenants, 75, 82–85;
the dialectic of the unwell and the
phenomenology of medicine,
66–81; and disease, 70–71; and
empathy, 65; and history of medical technology, 76–77; and illness,
68–69, 87n24, 87n26; infinity and
finitude, 61, 69–70, 78–79, 84–85;
and medical consumerism, 79, 80;
and the medical-industrial complex, 78–80; and medicine as a

profession, 73–75; and medicine as craft, 72–73; and pain, 61–64; and paradoxes of health care, 60–61; and sickness, 64, 67–68; and social utilitarianism, 80–81; subjectivity and objectivity, 61, 64–66, 80, 83–84; and suffering, 61–64, 86n10; and sympathy, 65; and technological medicine, 75–80; and the transcendent dimension of the human person, 63, 82–85; universality and particularity, 60–61, 70, 79, 80–81, 82–83; and unwellness, 67, 87n22; and the Witch Doctor, 71–72

Dickinson, Emily, 3–6, 8–9

difficult patients, caring for, 41–42

dignity: Aquinas on, 27–28; attributed, 32–33, 200–203, 210, 219–20; control and, 31; death-with-dignity discussions, 199–201; and Edson's *W;t*, 219–20; freedom and, 28, 29, 31–32; in Greco-Roman philosophy, 27; history of concept in Western thought, 25–29; and Hobbes, 28–29; and illness, 33; intrinsic, 29–33, 39–40, 200–203, 210, 219–20; and Kant, 28–29; in the Renaissance, 28; and Scripture, 26; and spiritual issues in the care of dying persons, 199–203, 210; and vulnerability of the healer, 39–40

Dillard, Annie, 195

disease: and the dialectic of healing, 70–71; as disturbance of right relationships, 125; technological medicine's focus on objective elements in, 80

Doctor–Priest Model, 176–78

Donne, John: and Edson's *W;t*, 215–16, 217; Holy Sonnet V, 215–16; "A Hymn to God the Father,"

207–9; and "Salvation Anxiety," 217

"do not resuscitate" (DNR) orders, 129, 189, 219

economic reconstruction of health care, 20–22

Emmaus story (Gospel of Luke), 19–20

empathy, 65

empirical research on spirituality in health care, 113–14, 115–20; association and causation, 117; caveats regarding, 115–20; intercessory prayer data, 118; and the naturalistic fallacy, 116–17, 120n1, 164; and outcomes data, 119–20, 152–54, 164–65, 182; quantification of the infinite, 118–19. *See also* biopsychosocial-spiritual model of health care; ethical issues regarding spirituality in health care; prayer, empirical studies of the healing power of

Engel, George, 122

The Enigma of Health (Gadamer), 9

Enlightenment medicine, 76

Essenes, 48–49

ethical issues regarding spirituality in health care, 161–85; charlatanism, 172–73, 178; and the collaborative model, 180–81, 182–83; and common justifications for addressing spirituality, 163–66; and consumer demand (patient requests), 165–66; and distortion of fourfold notion of patient's good, 181–82; the Doctor–Priest Model, 176–78; ethics, defining, 163; giving offense, 171–72; and imbalances of power, 181; issue of encouraging religious practice for health benefits, 181–82; and moral permissa-

ethical issues regarding spirituality in health care (*continued*) bility/moral duty, 163; the moral warrant to address spiritual issues, 167–69; and nonbelieving medical practitioners, 175–76; objections to introducing spirituality, 169–76; and outcomes data, 164–65; the parallel track model, 178–80, 182; and patients who profess no spiritual or religious beliefs, 173; and physicians' oaths, 168; and potential harm to patients, 173–75; religion/spirituality, defining, 162–63; and religious guilt, 174–75, 185n13; and religious patients who become sicker, 173; and spirituality as intrinsic to health care, 166–67. *See also* oaths, physicians'

European Middle Ages and Judeo-Christian understanding of medicine, 75–76

Exodus, book of, 53–57

FACIT-SP, 133

Fetzer Institute/National Institute on Aging Working Group, 130

Flexner, Abraham, 93, 98

Foucault's clinic, xi–xiii, 76, 77, 78, 179

French Revolution, xii, xvi

Freyer, David, 224

Gadamer, Hans-Georg, 9–11

George, Linda K., 138

Greco-Roman philosophy, 27

Greek medicine: and influence on Jewish medicine, 47–48, 49–50, 52, 75; rational approach and medicine as craft, 72–73; *therapeia*, 11

Hall, Donald, 201–2

Harris, William, and study of intercessory prayer, 147, 152, 153, 154

Havel, Vaclav, 205

Herth Hope Index, 135

Heschel, Abraham, 16

Hillel, 55

Hippocrates the Asclepiad, 9

Hippocratic Oath: alternatives for restoring Hippocratic oath-taking tradition, 104–5; and contemporary critics of Hippocratic ethics, 101; content of original, 104; and Jewish medicine, 50; and medicine as both science and art, 74; and medicine as profession, 73–75; Modified, 91–92, 96; professionalism and transcendence, 93, 97; as rite of passage, 92–93; as spiritual act, 92–93; trends to dispense with or replace, 79, 101. *See also* oaths, physicians'

Hobbes, Thomas, 28–29, 30

Holland, Jimmie, 225, 232

hospice movement, 224

Illich, Ivan, xii

illness: and "Deuteronomic retribution," 52–53; as disturbance of relationships, 125–26; and moral warrant to address spiritual issues, 168, 169; as objective recognition of the sick person's experience, 68–69, 87n24, 87n26; as spiritual event, 17; spiritual questions of, 166–67

industrialization of health care, 21

infinity and finitude: brought into opposition by illness, 69–70; caveats about quantifying, 118–19; as paradox of health care, 61; technology and healing, 78–79

INSPIRIT, 132

Institute of Noetic Sciences, 154
integrative medicine, xii
intercessory prayer. *See* prayer, empirical studies of the healing power of
International Code of Medical Ethics, 96

Jeral, Joseph M., 151–52, 156
Jewish medicine and medical ethics, 48–51; Babylonian influences, 49; Egyptian influences, 49–50; Essenes and Qumran community, 48–49; Greek/Hellenistic influences, 47–48, 49–50, 52, 75; Jewish innovations, 50–51; before time of Ben Sira, 48–49. *See also* Ben Sira, the Wisdom of
John Paul II, Pope, 62
Jonas, Hans, 125

Kant, Immanuel, 28–29, 90
Kenyon, Jane, 201–2, 205–6
King, Martin Luther, Jr., 30, 31, 200
Knight, Sara J., 133

Lonergan, Bernard, 190
love for patients, 34–35, 38
Luke's Gospel, the Emmaus story, 19–20

Maccabean revolt (166 BCE), 47
magic and healing, 51
Maimonides, 51
May, William, 56, 87n26
McGill Quality of Life Questionnaire, 133
Meaning in Life Scale, 133
medical school admissions, 106–7
Memorial Sloan Kettering Cancer Center, 233
miracles, 189–96; answering skeptics' arguments regarding, 189–92; in the Catechism of the Catholic Church, 192; and distinction between natural and supernatural, 190; and petitional prayer, 193–96; as revelations from God, 192–93; and scientific laws, 191; and secondary causation, 190
Moadel, Alyson, 133
molecular medicine, 77, 83
Moses, 53
Mytko, Johanna J., 133

National Institutes of Health (NIH), 154
naturalistic fallacy, 116–17, 120n1, 164
Nichomachean Ethics (Aristotle), 27

Oath of Asaph, 51
Oath of Dr. Louis Lasagna, 96
oaths, physicians', 89–112; alternatives for restoring oath-taking tradition, 104–5; arguments about moral irrelevance of, 89, 94–95, 101–3; concrete implications of taking seriously, 106–8; and courses in ethics and virtue, 107–8; and creation of a universal medical ethic, 105–6; and critics of Hippocratic ethics, 101; essential moral content of, 104–6; and the ethics of virtue, 96–97, 105; and Jewish medicine, 50; and medical school admissions, 106–7; and medicine as a profession, 73–75; and medicine as both science and art, 74; Modified Oath of Hippocrates, 91–92, 96; and moral warrant to address spiritual issues, 168; moral work involved in, 95–96; oaths and promises, defining, 90–91; original Hippocratic Oath, 104; patients' views of, 94–95; and professionalism, 93–94, 97, 98–101; and professional-

oaths, physicians' (*continued*)
ism, attacks on, 98–101; and
professionals' higher moral standard, 98–100; reasons for not
abandoning, 102–3; and right to
strike/perform work actions, 108;
as rite of passage, 92–93; as spiritual act, 92–93; and state medical
boards, 94–95; variety in common
use, 96; and White Coat ceremonies, 107. *See also* profession of
medicine
objectivity and subjectivity, 61, 64–
66, 80, 83–84
"On the Dignity of Man" (Pico della
Mirandola), 28
outcomes data: alternative ways of
dealing with, 152–54; caveats
about, 119–20; and empirical
studies of intercessory prayer,
152–54; and ethics of encouraging
patients to religious practice, 182;
as justification for addressing spirituality in health care, 164–65

pain, 61–64; differences between suffering and, 61–63; pain thresholds,
62
palliative care movement, 224
Parable of the Good Samaritan, 65
paradoxes in health care, 60–61; infinite and finite, 61; subjective and
objective, 61; universal and particular, 60–61
parallel track model, 178–80, 182
Parapsychology Foundation, 154
Pellegrino, Edmund D., 168, 181
Percival, Thomas, 204
Phaedrus (Plato), 9
physician-assisted suicide, 200
Pico della Mirandola, 28
Plato, 9
prayer, empirical studies of the healing power of, 147–60; Byrd study,

147, 152, 153, 154; caveats regarding data, 118; evaluating for
sources of bias, 154; Harris et al.
study, 147, 152, 153, 154; and
misplaced scientific critiques of
prayer, 157–58; moral critique of
studies, 155; operationalizing
prayer as an experimental intervention, 151–52; outcome measurements and statistical
problems, 152–54; randomization
and blinding, 148–51; sample size,
154; scientific critique of studies,
148–55; Sicher et al. study, 147,
149–50, 151, 152, 153, 154; and
studies showing longevity of people who attend religious services,
157–58; theological critique of
randomized trials, 155–57; Walker
et al. study, 147, 154
prayer, petitional, 193–96. *See also*
miracles
Prayer of Maimonides, 96
profession of medicine: and attacks
on professionalism, 98–101; and
Flexner's characteristics of a profession, 93–94; and moral warrant
to address spiritual issues, 168;
and a new spiritual interpretation
of health care, 83; and the phenomenology of medicine, 73–75;
and physicians' oaths, 73–75, 93–
94, 98–101; and role-specific
moral standards, 100–101; self-
regulation and standards/organiza-
tions, 108; and the transcendent
meaning of medicine, 93, 97. *See
also* oaths, physicians'
promises and oaths, 90–91
Ptolemy I of Egypt, 47
Puchalski, Christina M., 133

Rahner, Karl, 62
Ramsey, Paul, 18, 56, 63

Rawls, John, 81
RCOPE, 132
reconciliation: and forgiveness, 215–16, 221–22; and questions of relationship, 206–9, 211; and spiritual issues in the care of dying persons, 206–9, 211, 215–16
regenerative medicine, xii
religion: defining, 13–16, 124, 162–63; measuring religiosity, 130–31; measuring religious coping and support, 132. *See also* spirituality
Relman, Arnold, 78
Remen, Rachel, 137
Renaissance, 28
Ross, W. D., 90

Sausolito Consciousness Research Laboratory, 154
Schweitzer, Albert, 6
scientific reductionism, 21
Scripture: concept of human dignity in, 26; Jewish wisdom literature, 47–48. *See also* Ben Sira, the Wisdom of
Seleucus, 47
Sibyl of Cumae, 79
Sicher, Fred, and study of intercessory prayer, 147, 149–50, 151, 152, 153, 154
sickness, 64, 67–68
Simon Magus, 156
Sloan, Richard, 157, 158
Sokolowski, Robert, 64
somatization disorder, 87n24
spirituality: defining, 13–16, 124, 162–63; measuring the spiritual, 129–30, 132–33; problematic recent relationship between health care and, 16–17. *See also* religion
Spiritual Well-Being Scale, 133
Stoics, 27

subjectivity and objectivity, 61, 64–66, 80, 83–84
suffering, 61–64; differences between pain and, 61–63; and the experience of finitude, 63–64; a person as a being-in-relationship to others, 63, 64–65; philosophical anthropology of, 62–64, 86n10; responses to, 64–66; technological medicine and subjectivity of, 80; and the transcendent dimension of the human person, 63
Summa Theologiae (Thomas Aquinas), 27
sympathy, 65

Talmud, 45, 51
technological medicine, 75–80; and Enlightenment, 76; and European Middle Ages, 75–76; and finitude/infinitude, 78–79; and history of medical technology, 76–77; and medical consumerism, 79, 80; and the medical-industrial complex, 78–80; and molecular medicine, 77, 83; and objective elements of disease, 80; specialization and objective detachment in, 77, 79
Teilhard de Chardin, Pierre, 127
therapy (Greek *therapeia*), 11
Thomasma, David C., 181
touch, 17–18
transcendence and the human person, 18, 63; and new spiritual interpretation of health care, 82–85; and physicians' oaths and professionalism, 93, 97

unwellness: as deviations from homeostasis, 67, 87n22; and the phenomenology of medicine, 66–81
utilitarianism, 80–81, 102–3

vulnerability: of the healer, 38–40; and intrinsic dignity, 33–34,

39–40; and love for patients, 34–
35, 38; responding to, 34–38, 40

Walker, Scott, and study of interces-
sory prayer, 147, 154
Weil, Simone, 202–3
White, Kerr, 122
White Coat ceremonies, 107
Wisdom literature, 45. *See also* Ben
Sira, the Wisdom of
Wittgenstein, Ludwig, 15

World Health Organization (WHO),
132
W;t (Edson), 213–23, 226; dignity
theme, 219–20; and Donne's sonnets, 215–16, 217; and forgiveness, 215–16, 221–22; lessons for
clinicians, 220–21; reconciliation
theme, 215–16, 221–22; relationship theme, 217–19; themes receiving little attention from the
medical community, 213–14